PLACEBOS

PLACEBOS

KATHRYN T. HALL

The MIT Press | Cambridge, Massachusetts | London, England

The MIT Press would like to thank the anonymous peer reviewers who provided comments on drafts of this book. The generous work of academic experts is essential for establishing the authority and quality of our publications. We acknowledge with gratitude the contributions of these otherwise uncredited readers.

This book was set in Chaparral Pro by New Best-set Typesetters Ltd. Printed and bound in the United States of America.

Library of Congress Cataloging-in-Publication Data

Names: Hall, Kathryn T. (Kathryn Tayo) author.
Title: Placebos / Kathryn T. Hall.
Other titles: MIT Press essential knowledge series
Description: Cambridge, Massachusetts : The MIT Press, [2022] | Series: MIT Press essential knowledge series | Includes bibliographical references and index.
Identifiers: LCCN 2022000952 (print) | LCCN 2022000953 (ebook) | ISBN 9780262544252 (paperback) | ISBN 9780262371018 (pdf) | ISBN 9780262371025 (ebook)
Subjects: MESH: Placebos | Placebo Effect
Classification: LCC RM331 (print) | LCC RM331 (ebook) | NLM WB 330 | DDC 615.5—dc23/eng/20220511
LC record available at https://lccn.loc.gov/2022000952
LC ebook record available at https://lccn.loc.gov/2022000953

10   9   8   7   6   5   4   3   2   1

CONTENTS

SERIES FOREWORD

The MIT Press Essential Knowledge series offers accessible, concise, beautifully produced pocket-size books on topics of current interest. Written by leading thinkers, the books in this series deliver expert overviews of subjects that range from the cultural and the historical to the scientific and the technical.

In today's era of instant information gratification, we have ready access to opinions, rationalizations, and superficial descriptions. Much harder to come by is the foundational knowledge that informs a principled understanding of the world. Essential Knowledge books fill that need. Synthesizing specialized subject matter for nonspecialists and engaging critical topics through fundamentals, each of these compact volumes offers readers a point of access to complex ideas.

INTRODUCTION: THE BACK DOOR

It was a year and counting since the pain in my right wrist had taken me down that slippery slope from Advil to codeine. "Carpal tunnel syndrome" proclaimed my primary care physician. And with that I joined the intrepid bench scientists and computer programmers with telltale beige wrist braces who despite the pain of every click, kept pipetting, kept coding. I was working in the pharmaceutical industry at the time and although I didn't get addicted to the array of pain meds on my bedside stand, they did make it hard to concentrate. Only when I arrived at what was for me the last resort, surgery, was I willing to abdicate the logic of relief. The incision in my transverse carpal ligament recommended by the surgeon made sense, but it was so permanent. As my colleague who was disappointed in his surgery observed, positive results were no guarantee.

I was in pain, I was exhausted, I had nothing to lose. I called the number of the acupuncturist that my old friend, who had a black belt in aikido, had emailed me months ago, with the words "Just try it!!!" punctuated by three exclamation points.

Sitting in the waiting room of the acupuncturist, I studied what looked like subway maps on the human body. The stations had strange names like TW14 or L11. A strong smoky smell created a peculiar mix of curiosity and inertia that kept me sitting there long enough for a small woman to emerge from a bloodred door and usher me in. She began by asking me what I ate and what I did for exercise. Then she asked to look at my tongue. "Mmm, mhmm," she nodded as she peered into my mouth. "Lie down," she motioned brusquely to the massage table. The dull-orange sheet was pilled but looked clean. I hesitantly reclined. Taking my hand in hers, she placed her fingers delicately on my pulse, continuing her soft affirmations. Whatever she was learning from my pulse was most certainly flawed by my growing discomfort. Suddenly she reached away from the table, and in one fluid motion swung around and stuck a needle into my fingertip. Then another and another. It was ridiculous and intriguing. The thought of it hurt, but I hardly felt a thing; I was pinned.

Just as I was getting accustomed to this thing called acupuncture, she asked me to turn on my side and then she got up on the table. The shock of her hovering over me was no match for the pain that was about to come. She measured the back of my upper arm in finger lengths, and then finding a region around the middle, she palpated in closing circles till she found what she was looking for and again without notice, stuck in the needle. The burning was immediate and hot. "Aaahhh!" A sound both guttural and high-pitched, dragged from me involuntarily as the pain of the past year gathered together to make one last point. She twisted the needle, and another wave of heat and burn fired up and out my arm. As she made her way off the table, I was momentarily distracted by her descent. She was an older woman, of small stature, and very nimble. When I returned my focus to the matter at hand, I felt for the familiar pain in my wrist. It was gone. A year's struggle, gone. I searched my arm, my elbow, my wrist for the pain. Nothing.

She deftly placed several more needles across my body, now supine, and left me alone for some twenty minutes. Laying there I got used to the needles, some stuck in those same subway stops I had studied in the waiting room. Just as I was drifting off, she reappeared, rattling off a series of stern instructions. "Drink a lot more water, especially today," she said, casually pulling out needles from across my body. "Eat no red meat, do not drink alcohol, take a teaspoon of apple cider vinegar and honey every day." She wrapped her thin left hand over her right arm and pressed on a point at the center of the back of her arm. "If the pain returns, just rub this spot on the back of your arm, right here." She motioned for me to get up off the table. "OK, come back in two weeks." And with these few precepts, she showed me out the red door.

Returning to the safety of my car, I glanced at the discarded beige wrist support, waiting patiently on the passenger seat. I wriggled my fingers, flexed, and then rotated my wrist. Still nothing, no pain. Deeply relieved and totally perplexed, I drove back to work that afternoon. I was an associate director of drug development at a biopharmaceutical company. I was headed back to the heart of biotech in Cambridge, Massachusetts. Over the years, when the pain in my wrist would return, I massaged that same spot, and sure enough, the pain would dissipate. I would contemplate the how and why of that clinical encounter for years to come. Why did that work? Was it the power of acupuncture or *just* a placebo effect?

Acupuncture is an ancient healing tradition. Honed over centuries, the theories behind acupuncture are complex and elegant. Of the complementary and alternative medicines, now termed *integrative medicine*, studied in the United States, acupuncture has demonstrated the greatest efficacy in treating pain. Sham acupuncture can also elicit strong placebo responses. Sham acupuncture needles are designed like a trick sword; instead of the needle penetrating the skin, it disappears into a shaft. Clinical trials of acupuncture often find similar effects between acupuncture performed with real needles compared to placebo or sham needles.[1]

Placebos, like sham acupuncture needles, are inert simulacra of active drugs, devices, or other treatments. However inert a treatment may be, placebos and their administration can have striking ameliorative properties. When the administration of inert treatment leads to a clinical benefit, it is called a *placebo effect*. Even though the placebo interventions themselves have no biological qualities that would induce a physiological change, placebo effects can be long-lasting and are at times competitive with the clinical benefits of active treatments. Herein lies the placebo's paradox, which has puzzled and provoked researchers and clinicians for centuries—that is, until the underlying mechanisms began to emerge.

Acupuncture is not alone in inducing a robust placebo response. The administration of the placebo form of many Western therapies and even surgery can bring about powerful placebo effects. In fact, pharmaceutical drug development, particularly the development of novel drugs in neurological and psychological disease areas, is finding it increasingly difficult to demonstrate efficacy beyond that of a placebo. And it's not just drugs; some sham surgeries were found to be as beneficial as the well-established surgical procedures they were being compared to. Why does this happen? And importantly, what does this mean for medicine, especially Western medicine, and healing in the present day? Does the placebo effect tell us something about how human beings heal? And therefore how we, as scientists and clinicians, approach our research and patients?

This book is not about whether acupuncture, Western medicine, or surgery works. It is about neurobiological mechanisms that influence almost every clinical encounter we engage in, regardless of whether the treatment is active or inert. Throughout this book, we learn of the power of these underlying mechanisms, and my goal is to examine the intentional and unintentional uses of placebos in the past and present, and how they have benefited or harmed people whose lives they touched.

The word *placebo* comes from the Latin "I shall please" and was used to describe hired mourners in the fourteenth century who were paid to simulate mourning at the funerals of those who could afford it.[2] These hired mourners were nicknamed placebos after their characteristic chant "Placebo Domino in regione vivorum," I will please the Lord in the land of the living. In this early iteration of the placebo, these mourners aided the process of grieving, giving permission to those in attendance to give way to whatever emotions might need catharsis. Even though placebos functioned to support a psychological process necessary to the human psyche, they were considered to be fake and negatively associated with death. Geoffrey Chaucer reinforced this negative connotation by naming the sycophant in the *Merchant's Tale* Placebo.

Despite these negative undertones, placebos would make their way into medical vernacular through the writings of William Cullen, one of the most influential physicians in the eighteenth century. This is where I pick up the story of placebos in chapter 1, "Placebos: A Brief History." In this chapter, I examine how placebos were ensnared by quackery and patent medicine, and emerged as controls in clinical trials.

Patent or proprietary medicines were remedies marketed and sold directly to consumers without any regulatory approval. The most powerful attribute of these nostrums was not their contents, which were often inert and at times harmful, but instead their trademarked names. From "Mrs. Winslow's Soothing Syrup" and "Dr. Sawen's Magic Nervine Pills" to "Lydia E. Pinkham's Vegetable Compound" and "Dr. J. W. Coblenz's No. 1 Tonic," there was a patent medicine for just about everything. The power of a trademark, and information to drive the experience and perceived benefit of a treatment, was not lost in the development of modern-day drug manufacturers that continue to shape expectations of the clinical benefits through the packaging, names, and advertisements of therapies.[3]

Our expectations are informed by our personal experience, the observed experiences of others, and cues and symbols, through which associative learning or conditioning can guide our expectations for a given outcome. Expectations and associative learning are critical drivers of a response to placebos, and I explore their effects in chapter 2, "How Expectations and Conditioning Shape Placebo Effects."

The idea that inert, sham, or placebo interventions can induce neurobiological effects that in turn promote positive clinical outcomes may appear to be paradoxical to our mechanistic understanding of the cause and treatment of disease. But is it? In chapter 3, "The Brain on Placebos," I look at the amazing developments in neuroimaging that are revealing the inner workings of placebo effects. I will track the neurobiological changes that are induced by placebo treatment in experimental studies of analgesia in healthy participants. I will also briefly discuss the neurobiological correlates of the placebo effect in patients with Parkinson's disease and depression, demonstrating that we are hardwired to override a modicum of pain and suffering. The hardwired neurobiological mechanisms at the heart of placebo effects are not limited to placebos. They have been observed in the many situations in which our expectations rewrite our perception and even experience of incoming information. In this way, these mechanisms represent a back door to enhancing both wellness and suffering.

Why have we evolved to be sensitive to expectation and placebo effects? Medical historians and physicians are fond of saying that early medicines were all placebos. That may be so, but if it has taken until now for effective drugs to be made, how did we survive the pain and suffering of primitive times? Surely survival of the fittest meant survival of those who could overcome and manage bodily hurt and harm?[4] Historical records tell us that as we evolved, we assigned trusted people in the community to know and recall which plants and animals in our environment were beneficial to our health. Over time, these shamans, *sangomas*, *mudangs*, *curanderos*, and *curanderas* developed tried-and-true rituals and symbols that accompanied the dispensation of these remedies, cultivating in human societies a link between the act of treatment and the neurobiological mechanisms that override pain and suffering.

Today, nowhere is this more powerfully demonstrated than in the clinical encounter in the proverbial doctor's office. There, symbols include not only the mise-en-scène-—the stethoscope, white coat, and exam table—but also the ritual and practice of the doctor visit. Think about it: from the moment we are born, many of us enter into a room of masked people in scrubs or white coats; we are literally in the hands of medicine. What follows for many of us is years of associative learning and conditioning. Reinforced by our parents, we learn to return to the doctor's office when we are unwell, or for checkups and disease preventive vaccinations. If we have positive or at least beneficial experiences, we build an expectation that though the pills will be bitter and the vaccination might hurt, these interventions will protect us from or cure disease. No matter the treatment, if administered with care and confidence, and if we are not afflicted by infectious diseases or cancer that operate outside our command, we have a good chance of feeling better.

Expectation and conditioning promote placebo effects, but they can induce negative or nocebo effects as well. From COVID-19 vaccination resistance to reluctance to use statins in cardiovascular disease prevention, negative information can have adverse effects on the individual, and therefore collectively have detrimental impacts on public health. In chapter 4, "Nocebo Effects in Modern Medicine," I discuss this so-called opposite of the placebo effect in medicine and popular culture. In this book, I argue, as many others have, that the neurobiological mechanisms that mediate expectation and drive placebo and nocebo effects can enhance the benefits of treatment, but also make us vulnerable. Thus we see that this mechanism can be co-opted for better or worse.

For the last seventy-five years, placebos have played a pivotal role as controls in clinical trials. As controls, placebos work best when used in studies of diseases in which a placebo response has little clinical benefit. For the most part, these are trials of cellular (cancer), viral (COVID-19), or bacterial (pneumonia) proliferation, where belief or expectation can do little to fight the spread of the disease. Although placebo effects appear to have little impact on the outcome of these trials, it's important to note that it's not that patients enrolled in cancer, antiviral, or antibacterial trials are not having a placebo response. Rather, the biological pathway stimulated by placebo effects is no match for these diseases. In neurological, psychological, and some cardiovascular conditions like hypertension, however, the placebo-targeted biological pathways can have real and durable effects. Further, there is growing evidence that genes and drugs can independently and combinatorially influence a placebo response in clinical trials. In chapter 5, "Placebos in Clinical Trials," I look at the role of placebo controls in randomized clinical trials of pharmaceuticals and the challenges of demonstrating efficacy beyond a placebo in conditions characterized by high rates of placebo responses.

Recently, placebo or sham surgeries have demonstrated remarkably positive effects in the placebo or control treatment arms for well-established surgeries. In chapter 6, "The Placebo Effect in Surgery," I examine the use of sham surgery as a control and discuss how present-day findings are influencing our belief in the efficacy of some surgeries. Improving clinical trials relies on being able to predict placebo responders so we can harness and manage placebo effects. In chapter 7, I explore the question of "Who Responds?" to placebos, and take a look at what psychology and genetics tell us about predicting placebo responders.

And finally, in chapter 8, "Placebo Redux," I focus on the role placebos are playing in current times, and the new challenges and opportunities provided by technological advances like virtual reality, artificial intelligence, and digital therapeutics, termed *digiceuticals*.

Placebos are a back door to one of our most valuable assets: our health. In hacker terms, a *back door* is a hidden entrance that can provide access to manipulate and

Placebos are a back door to one of our most valuable assets: our health.

establish control of a network. As neuroimaging studies bring the mechanisms of the action of placebos into clear view, we are learning that there are regions in the brain that can be induced, through expectations, to override the networks that process incoming sensations of pain or other symptoms. Variously championed by well-meaning healers and assaulted by quacks, the access that placebos offer to our health and well-being has been hiding in plain sight. Only now as the levers of the powerful placebo are being revealed are we in a position to understand our individual and collective roles and responsibilities. Surely it is incumbent on us to safeguard and use the power of placebos for good.

PLACEBOS

A Brief History

Two pieces of wood, properly shaped and painted, were next made use of. . . . In four minutes, the man raised his hand several inches, and he had lost also the pain in his shoulder usually experienced when attempting to lift anything. He continued to undergo the operation daily, and with progressive good effect; for on the 25th he could touch the mantle-piece.

This patient at length so far recovered, that he could carry coals and use his arm sufficiently to assist the nurse; yet previous to the use of the spurious Tractors he could no more lift his hand from his knee than if a hundred weight were upon it, or a nail driven through it. . . . The fame of this case brought applications in abundance; indeed, it must be confessed, that it was more than sufficient to act

> upon weak minds, and induce a belief that these
> pieces of wood and iron were endowed with some
> peculiar virtues.
>
> —John Haygarth, *Of the Imagination*, January 1, 1800

It was New Year's Day, 1800, and Haygarth, a noted physician and student of William Cullen, famed first physician to the king of Scotland, had an axe to grind.[1] On retiring to Bath after a brilliant career in medicine, Haygarth had grown increasingly appalled at the popularity among the wealthy elite of two small handheld devices touted to have extraordinary curative powers.[2] Known as Perkins's tractors, the metallic rods were a US import. By simply drawing the tractors over an afflicted body part, Elisha Perkins, their inventor, claimed to be able to remove rheumatism, gouty affections, pleurisies, inflammation, epileptic fits, lockjaw, and pain and swelling from contusions, sprains, burns, and headaches. Not even Haygarth, who would put the tractors to the test, could dispute their effectiveness.

Perkins (1741–1799) was a Yale-trained physician who was himself the son of a physician. During oral surgeries, he observed that contact with metal could induce focal analgesia and make muscles contract. He fashioned a pair of three-inch metal rods to see if they might have a curative effect on his patients. His early tests were so positive that he took out a patent, and as was the custom of the day, named the invention after himself. Perkins and his Perkins Patent Tractors gained rapid popularity (figure 1). The rods were rounded at one end and sharpened at the apex; one was made of silver and platinum, and the other was made of copper, zinc, and gold. They cost only a shilling to make and sold for a whopping five guineas (around five hundred dollars) a pair. Buoyed by his success, he presented his invention at the Connecticut Medical Society meeting of 1795, ascribing the tractors' healing powers to galvanism and the newly discovered therapeutic effects of electric currents. Perkins was greeted with derision and a wall of skepticism and soon after left Connecticut, taking his invention to Philadelphia, the then US capital, where Congress was in session. There the tractors continued to grow in popularity. George Washington purchased a pair, and the Honorable Oliver Ellsworth, former chief justice of the Supreme Court, wrote to the Honorable John Marshall, the sitting chief justice, remarking, "The effects wrought are not easily ascribed to imagination, great and delusive as is its power." But Perkins's personal success would be short-lived. When yellow fever broke out in New York City, Perkins claimed to have discovered the cure. In 1799, armed with a tincture of vinegar and muriate of soda, he headed to New York. There he feverishly administered his antiseptic for four weeks before he himself contracted the virus and died. By the time of Perkins's death, however, the tractors were well on their way to the elite summer circles in Bath.

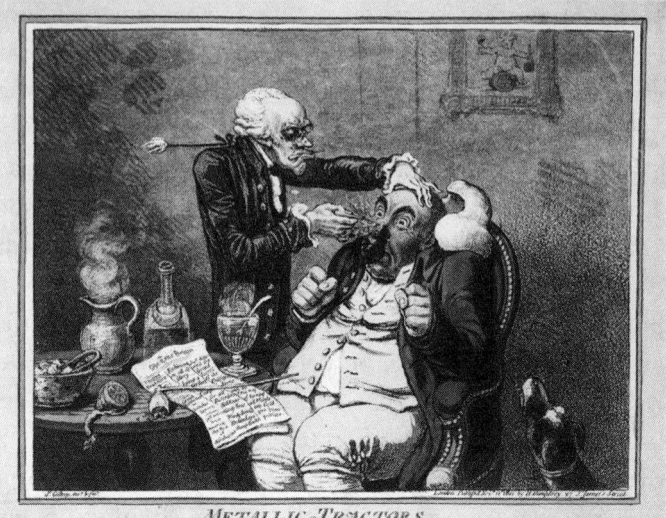

Figure 1 Cartoon sketch by James Gillray, 1801, of a quack treating a patient with Perkins Patent Tractors.

Haygarth was a man of reason. His advocacy of smallpox vaccines is credited with reducing the spread of the disease in late eighteenth-century Great Britain. As a student of Cullen, Haygarth would likely have been familiar with the great physician's teachings on use of a "pure placebo" (a bread or sugar pill), or lower doses of regular drugs to please, palliate, or "give what might be of use to the patient."[3] But palliative placebos administered by caring physicians were one thing; patent medicines like Perkins's tractors were entirely something else. As Haygarth wrote, the tractors, having "obtained such a high reputation at Bath, even among persons of rank and understanding," required the discerning attention of physicians.[4]

In deciding on a process to investigate the tractors, Haygarth had a compelling precedent. Just over a decade earlier in 1784, an all-too-similar outbreak of marginal science had infiltrated elite Parisian circles. The inventor was Franz Anton Mesmer, a successful Austrian physician. Having used magnets to cure a young woman of a host of maladies including fevers, vomiting, toothaches, and intermittent paralysis, Mesmer hypothesized that a fluid, which he named animal magnetism, penetrated and encircled all bodies, and could be used to heal patients. Mesmer and mesmerism, as his technique came to be called, gained fame and fortune as he wielded a large metal rod over patients to move the fluid in the service of healing. At the time, Mesmer's techniques and their apparent theatrics gripped even the upper echelons of French society. Demand grew, and he scaled up his operation with the invention of a "baquet," a large oak tub filled with "magnetized" water from which iron rods protruded. Scores of patients encircled the baquet, gripping the iron rods, pressing against each other to allow the magnetic fluid to flow. As incense and empyrean tones wafted through the air, patrons would fall into "crises" resembling violent convulsions. Piercing shrieks or bouts of laughter erupted as the patients juddered back to health. Despite the fact that his wife, Marie Antoinette, was a frequent baquet flyer, or perhaps because of it, King Louis XVI yielded to pressure from the medical establishment to investigate Mesmer.

To lead his Royal Commission on the danger to the public morals posed by "animal magnetism," Louis XVI tapped the distinguished and beloved US ambassador to the French court, Benjamin Franklin. Franklin was joined by an all-star team of distinguished scientists including Antoine Lavosier, the "father of chemistry," Jean-Sylvain Bailly, a famous astronomer, and the physician Joseph-Ignace Guillotin, who also happened to be a strong proponent of the rapid decapitation device that later would bear his name.[5] While the Royal Commission claimed its sole interest was evaluating animal magnetism, its commentary as it started its investigations suggested that there were deep concerns that should the practice of magnetism take hold, "the whole science of medicine would become useless." The commissioners spent three to four months conducting what might be considered one of the first clinical trials. Franklin hosted some of the simulated sessions at his home in Passy. At Franklin's lead, the commission created sham mesmerized rods and water. He had imposters pose as practitioners. They witnessed firsthand the crises wrought as their placebo controls incited the same group dynamics that the true mesmerists induced: participants convulsed, retched, and screamed—sometimes for hours. In the final analysis, Franklin and the commission concluded that while mesmerism did indeed elicit the striking effects for which it had become known, the same effects were induced with fake objects and sham practitioners.

Haygarth versus Perkins: Another Early Clinical Trial

Franklin died in 1785, some years before Haygarth launched his investigation into Perkins's tractors. But it's easy to see Franklin's influence on Haygarth in the use of sham devices as controls in his tractor trial. Haygarth was well acquainted with Franklin and his work. The two men had corresponded by mail, with Haygarth sharing guidance on how inoculations could prevent the spread of smallpox in the United States. Franklin's second son, Franky, had succumbed to smallpox at the age of four, making Franklin a strong proponent of inoculations to stem the spread of the disease. So much so that in his autobiography, Franklin is famous for lamenting that he "long regretted that [he] had not given it to him [Franky] by Inoculation."[6] Haygarth was likely also influenced by Arthur Lee, a protégé of Franklin whose help he enlisted in designing the Perkins's trial. Lee was likely familiar with the dummy rods and sham mesmerists that Franklin employed to test whether animal magnetism really worked.

Haygarth fashioned sham Perkins's tractors of wood, and painted them gold and silver so no one would be the wiser. He sent these out to other physicians with strict instructions that patients be unaware of the ruse. His 1800 manuscript detailing the results of this study, titled *Of the Imagination, as a Cause and as a Cure of Disorders of the Body; Exemplified by Fictitious Tractors and Epidemical Convulsions*, would be widely disseminated, rivaling the popularity of the tractors themselves.[7] The cases reported in the manuscript were and still are today nothing short of remarkable. Take, for instance, one Thomas Ellis, who was so severely afflicted with rheumatism that he was unable to walk without support or feed himself for months. On being treated with the wooden tractors, he felt his skin growing warmer with occasional darting pains and throbbing on a cicatrix. After ten days of sessions, he was able to comb his hair, put on his jacket, and walk across the ward without a stick or the least assistance. In this manner, patient after patient was restored to health. Thus, Franklin and Haygarth came to the same conclusion. Their key finding was not that these strange and bewildering remedies didn't work; it was that the sham devices worked just as well as the real ones.

Franklin and Haygarth came to the same conclusion: not that these strange remedies didn't work, but that the sham devices worked just as well as the real ones.

The efforts of Franklin and Haygarth to stem the growing popularity of nostrums and patent medicines would be in vain. Despite the discovery of the pathogenicity of microbes and disease preventive effects of pasteurization and vaccines in the mid-1800s, clinical objectivity would be slow to take hold. Another century of rampant quackery would pass before "regular" or "orthodox" physicians would gain enough power to curtail the charlatanry.

Integrative Medicine

Part of the popularity enjoyed by quacks in the nineteenth century was driven by fear of so-called regular physicians. *Regular* was the term given to physicians educated at university-affiliated medical colleges. They were classically trained to use heroic medicine—bleeding, sweating, and emetics—to shock the body back to health. With this limited approach, it is not surprising that the milder "irregular" physicians, including mesmerists (later renamed hypnotists), water cure specialists, and homeopaths, remained popular among the public. Many of these milder therapies had much to recommend them, and their popularity would endure into modern times. In various forms, some of these treatments—hypnosis, homeopathy, and hydrotherapy—are now practiced under the umbrella of integrative medicine.

Hypnosis, or the induction of a trancelike state in which the subject is highly responsive and susceptible to suggestion, is a commonly used therapeutic technique in the treatment of pain and psychological challenges, including anxiety, depression, and post-traumatic stress syndrome. The technique is thought to have partially been inspired by the theatrics of Mesmer and mesmerism and was briefly used in place of anesthesia for surgeries in the nineteenth century.[8] Much later, hypnosis re-emerged as a respected technique used among psychologists. In 1958, the American Medical Association (AMA) approved a report that stated that there were "definite and proper uses of hypnosis in medical and dental practice."[9] This support was later echoed by the American Psychiatric Association and a National Institutes of Health panel of experts, and the topic remains of interest among clinicians, social psychologists, and neuroscientists alike.

Founded by Samuel Hahnemann (1755–1843), homeopathic medicine is based on the "principle of similars": a condition can be cured with a treatment that induces in a healthy person the very symptoms that afflict a patient. This principle of "like cures like" was derived from Hahnemann's own experience inducing malarial symptoms of intermittent fever using bark from a cinchona tree, which, as it turns out, contains quinine. To minimize the toxic effects of some of his remedies, Hahnemann serially diluted the active agents in alcohol or water so that only a trace amount remained. Another notable feature of homeopathy is the typically hour-long consultation in which the patient's life and illness are painstakingly discussed. In part because of its beneficial effects and enduring popularity, homeopathy would survive into the modern era despite the reservations of physicians educated in Western medicine, who remained skeptical about the efficacy of the infinitesimal.[10]

Hydrotherapy, or the so-called water cure, was an alternative treatment method that originated from the belief that pure water had significant healing benefits. Hydrotherapists administered the cure, water, through a variety of routes: patients would drink large quantities of water, sit in cold baths and use douches, and/or rub wet bandages and sheets on the body, all in combination with exercise and a simple diet. What these milder irregular therapies have in common is likely the ability to induce strong placebo effects.[11] But not all therapies originating in this era were as benign.

Quacks, Charlatans, and Patent Medicine

Even clergy who had access to free care from regular physicians opted for irregular medicine techniques, including nostrums and tonics, lending their names and credibility to testimonials and advertisements, thereby reinforcing and driving the popularity of these treatments. Lumped in with the irregular physicians were the physician quacks. These were physicians who were either poorly trained or, as in the cases of Mesmer and Perkins, well trained only to go the way of proprietary medicine with an invention that exploited the placebo effect. There were also the quacks who claimed to be physicians, patenting or more precisely trademarking the name on the label as opposed to the formulation of the medicine. This was probably because patenting a product required disclosing its contents, and the contents of many, if not most, nostrums and tonics would have dissuaded any thoughtful consumer, as we will soon see.

Regular physicians were not allowed to advertise, and this put them at a tremendous disadvantage in relation to quacks who used flyers, magazines, religious and secular papers, and the press to appeal to sufferers of every ailment imaginable with an offer of a miraculous cure. The rise of medical societies and journals gave the regular physicians a platform from which to take aim at nostrums, quackery, and pseudomedicine. Regular physicians had already begun to consolidate their power during the American Civil War (1861–1865) by requiring medical examinations and degrees from proprietary medical schools for physicians to volunteer in the physician corps of the Union Army. Still in the 1800s, US patent medicines constituted 28 percent of marketed drugs.[12] Aided by advertisements to the unwitting public and many a physician, this would grow to 72 percent by 1900.

Some of the more effective remedies were far from placebos. One of the most popular and powerful of these was Mrs. Lydia E. Pinkham's Vegetable Compound, a women's tonic for menstrual and menopausal discomfort. This tonic was composed of a mixture of herbs including an extract from the Jamaica dogwood distilled in alcohol. The bark of the Jamaica dogwood (*Piscidia erythrina* or *Piscidia piscipula*) is used in traditional remedies to treat pain, insomnia, menstrual cramps, anxiety, and fear. The bark contains rotenone, a compound that kills fish by impeding respiration, and its use was banned in the Caribbean, where fishers would throw it in the water to stun fish. The bottle featured an image of Mrs. Pinkham, always in formal dress, and hair parted down the middle with a Mona Lisa smile (figure 2). Her advertising campaign would position her company as one of the most successful patent medicine companies of the late 1800s and beyond her death into the early 1900s. Frozen in time and looking as surprised to see her as we are, Mrs. Pinkham appears on the packaging of her Herbal Tablet Supplement available on Amazon today!

As residents of Lynn, Massachusetts, the Pinkhams tried to gain credibility by engaging nearby Harvard Medical School physicians to conduct a controlled study comparing the vegetable compound to a placebo control.[13] While

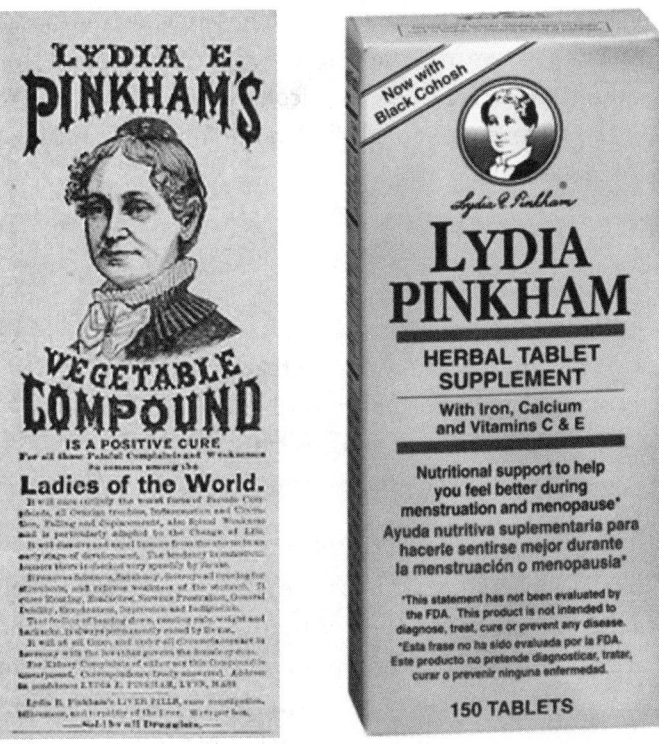

Figure 2 Labels from Lydia E. Pinkham's Vegetable Compound products, then (left) and now.

the Pinkhams wanted the researchers to use a water-based product as a control, the Harvard physicians argued that as the tonic was 18 percent alcohol, they would have to use the same amount of alcohol in the control. The studies were never done.

The Augean Stables

> When the veil of mystery is torn from the medical figure the naked sordidness and inherent worthlessness that remains suffices to make quackery its own greatest condemnation.
>
> —Samuel Smith, *The Great American Fraud*, 1905

Not all tonics and nostrums were as well conceived or well intended, and by the turn of the twentieth century, the harms, both financial and physical, were mounting. For the most part, quackery preyed on the hopes and desperation of an ailing public. The quack direct marketing process was simple. If you wrote a letter of inquiry in response to an ad, you would receive a seemingly personalized letter designed to build your expectations as well as convince you that the patent medicine was used to great effect by the inventor and other patients with symptoms similar to yours. These letters ended with the cost of the nostrums and a special deal, just for you, because the inventor was so concerned with your case. If you, as the potential patient, did not respond, another letter announcing a sudden fortuitous discount would be sent, and so on, until you, the prospective patient, took the bait and bought the mail-order treatment. There was little recourse after this; attempts to return ineffective or damaging treatments were met with complete disregard for the victim.

The press became dependent on the advertising money paid by patent medicine companies, and shied away from publishing reports that might draw attention to the damage being done to pocketbook and person. Because the US Postal Service was the mechanism by which letters, then money, and then goods were exchanged, not surprisingly it was the postmaster general working with the AMA that would eventually halt the flow of proprietary medicines.

To discourage the production of fake or harmful medications, the AMA started a voluntary drug validation program in 1905 that would remain a requirement until 1955. For drugs to obtain the AMA Seal of Acceptance and be advertised in the *Journal of the American Medical Association*, they had to be assessed by the AMA's Council on Pharmacy and Chemistry, proven to treat ailments as claimed, and shown to contain safe and high-quality ingredients. In 1905, the AMA also doubled down on quackery by republishing a series of articles by Samuel Smith that had appeared in *Collier's* magazine titled "The Great American Fraud," detailing the crimes and misdemeanors of "the nostrum evil and quackery." The series sold tens of thousands of copies. Each article detailed the US Department of Agriculture's chemical analysis of the patent medicine's contents and ensuing legal proceedings against the proprietors. What emerged was far from a benign story of placebo effects. While Dr. Turner's obesity cure was nothing but starch, ginger, talc, ash, and milk by-products, Dr. Curry's cancer cures contained antiseptics, hydrogen peroxide, and preparations of opium and cocaine. Perhaps the most vicious were the business concerns that peddled the very ingredients that were the sources of people's addictions. Dr. J. W. Coblenz was a case in point; his advertisements included a word of advice to the victim of morphine addiction that the way to conquer the habit was through persistence. All the while, the key ingredients in Coblenz's No. 1 tonic were alcohol and morphine. Similarly, Habitina, touted as a gradual reduction treatment for addiction to pain-alleviating and sleep-producing drugs that did not poison the system like plain "morphin," was in fact a combination of morphine and heroine that left the patients worse than they were before taking the treatment (figure 3). It is no wonder that placebos, ensnared in charlatanry, would take another hundred years to extricate themselves from this Augean stable.

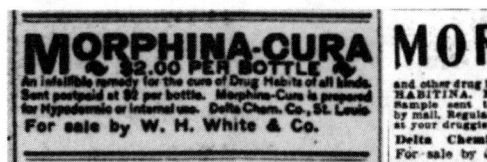

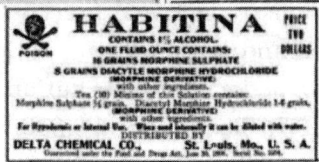

Figure 3 Habitina labels over time. Habitina was a patent medicine sold as a cure for addiction to morphine. When the US Food and Drug Administration required the disclosing of contents on the label, Habitina was revealed to have morphine as an ingredient.

Regulatory Affairs

In 1906, the Pure Food and Drugs Act was passed by Congress. The terms for "adulterated" and "misbranded" were finally delineated, opium and alcohol were classified as dangerous ingredients, and drug labels to indicate the presence of these compounds were required. While quacks were required to state the contents of their treatments, regular physicians ironically had no such requirement in the dispensation of placebos. Despite this apparent contradiction, Richard Cabot confirmed this continued ubiquity of placebos in medicine in his 1909 review of "Truth and Falsehood in Medicine": "I was brought up, as I suppose every physician is, to use what are called placebos, that is bread pills, subcutaneous injections of a few drops of water (supposed by the patient to be morphine), and other devices for acting on the patient's symptoms through his mind."[14]

It would take tragedy and an act of Congress to cement the US Food and Drug Administration's (FDA) control over the production and distribution of pharmaceutical drugs. In 1937, Elixir Sulfanilamide, marketed for treating a variety of infections from strep throat to gonorrhea, left seventy-one adults and thirty-four children dead. Far from a placebo, the formulation included a commonly used antibacterial agent, sulfanilamide, dissolved in a deadly proportion of diethylene glycol (antifreeze). The lethal events shocked physicians and legislators alike, and at long last hastened the confirmation of legally binding guidelines for drug production. In 1938, Congress finally implemented the Federal Food, Drug, and Cosmetic Act, introducing critical regulations on drug production and distribution, including proof of safety before distribution, and limits on the amount of poisonous matter in drug factories.

Emergence of Placebos as Controls in Clinical Trials

As the study of metabolism, physiology, and pharmacology were formalized as research disciplines in the 1920s and 1930s, the use of controls—especially placebos—in clinical studies became indispensable. When Harry Gold, a pharmacologist at Cornell University Medical College, began to investigate the use of xanthines to relieve cardiac pain in the 1930s, he was aware of the vagaries of placebo effects. He set about to screen out placebo responders by excluding patients who could not correctly attribute their pain relief to glyceryl trinitrate versus a soluble placebo taken under the tongue at the onset of an attack of pain. As many patients were unable to discern the difference between the drug and placebo, he was forced to abandon his screening effort. Gold enrolled one hundred patients who suffered from cardiovascular disease and heart pain in what would be one of the first n-of-1 studies in which the patients were their own controls, crossing over from xanthine to placebo and back throughout the course of the study. After five years, the study was completed in 1937 and found no difference between pain reduction with xanthine compared to the placebo. Impressed with the placebo effects in this and other studies, Gold, a pharmacologist, would become a strong proponent of the benefits of placebo therapy. By World War II, the use of placebos in blinded clinical trials would be well accepted, though randomization had not yet entered the equation.

In 1946, at the end of World War II, Gold joined Eugene Dubois and other scientists at the Conference on Therapy sponsored by Cornell University Medical College. This was the first conference where placebos were openly and actively discussed. But Gold's positive view that "the placebo is a specific psychotherapeutic device with values of its own" was met with opposition on ethical grounds. Henry Richardson, a psychiatrist from Peter Bent Brigham Hospital in Boston, summed up the ethical concerns: "I don't like the element of deception in a placebo, apart from the fact that it is disastrous to get found out. I think that if there is to be a deception it should be the one which the patient demands and which, also, I think he needs."[15] Again, the fault with placebos was not that they didn't work but instead that they were linked to deception and relegated to the unethical.

The Declaration of Helsinki, written to address ethical practices for clinical research, built on the Nuremberg Code of 1947 to address human experimentation and other human rights atrocities committed in the name of medical research in Germany during World War II. If there was any hope to use placebos deceptively in the clinic, the Declaration of Helsinki in 1964 shut the door. Though the declaration itself was not legally binding for physicians, it marked a shift in the general perception of physicians and medical ethics, and contributed to a variety of legislations that strongly influenced the future of human subject research. Modern ethical practices are generally derived from the 1978 Belmont Report along with the work of Thomas Beauchamp and James Childress, who introduced the central ethical principles of respect for autonomy, non-maleficence, beneficence, and justice. Importantly, these new tenets of clinical and experimental ethics prohibited any form of deception of the patient. This policy posed a problem for physicians who had taken to prescribing placebos to hard-to-treat patients. Because it was believed that the treatment would not work if patients knew they were being given inert treatments, the question of using placebos in clinical practice was a nonstarter. Although the randomized placebo-controlled clinical trial would become the gold standard for evaluating the efficacy of drugs, it would take over a half century for researchers to formally challenge the requirement of deception for placebos to work.[16]

The Powerful Placebo

Henry Beecher, born Harry Knowles Unangst in 1904, was intimately aware of the power of information to shape expectations and perceptions. After college, a master's degree in physical chemistry, and a name change, he left his home state of Kansas for the hallowed halls of Harvard Medical School. As Beecher, he graduated in 1932, and by 1941 was the first endowed chair in anesthesiology in the United States. When World War II broke out, Beecher served as an army physician on the front lines in North Africa and Italy. He witnessed firsthand how expectations of pain relief could ameliorate the suffering of soldiers wounded in battle, and on his return to Massachusetts General Hospital, focused his research on painkillers like morphine.[17] Beecher became fascinated with what he called placebo reactors: patients who responded to the placebo controls. Although he was not at the Cornell meeting in 1946, his landmark paper published in the *Journal of the American Medical Association* a decade later on Christmas Eve 1955 was a gift to the future of placebos. This modern formulation, fittingly titled "The Powerful Placebo," was a tour de force of all things placebo. Beecher discussed their utility as psychological instruments in mental illness, a treatment to be used by the harassed clinician of the neurotic patient, and controls to eliminate bias and help in determining the effects of drugs. He summarized several earlier findings by other groups that pointed to the power of placebos to activate biological processes including the adrenals (the fight-or-flight response) in much the same way a drug could, arguing that the effects of placebo highlight a fundamental common mechanism that warranted further serious investigation. In what would be considered an early meta-analysis, he determined that 35 percent of people across fifteen studies responded to placebos. Although some researchers debate his methods, his finding is certainly in the ballpark of what is seen today in trials of chronic and functional pain conditions. He also listed thirty-five side effects observed with placebo treatment and exhorted the use of placebo controls in assessing efficacy as well as side effects. Beecher asserted that placebo and drug effects were additive, suggesting that excluding placebo reactors from studies would boost the difference between drugs and placebos.

Research on Placebos

Experimentation on placebos would continue through the 1960s and 1970s. These studies explored the role of conditioning and expectation in response to inert treatments. Although endogenous opioids were suspected as mediators of a placebo response, it wasn't until Jon Levine and Howard Fields examined the influence of naloxone and opioid antagonists that there was confirmation of this hypothesis. They demonstrated that naloxone (trademarked as Narcan) blocked a placebo response after molar extraction, suggesting that opioid signaling might play a role in placebo responses.[18] This finding showed that placebo effects have an objective, biological basis and thus changed physician's impressions of the potential of placebos across the world. A new era of placebo research was about to begin.

Soon after, behavioral psychologists weighed in with theories of expectation and conditioning in the placebo effect. In 1985, Irving Kirsch posited that placebo responsiveness is a result of response expectancies that can affect experience, physiology, and behavior. Since then, there has been modest debate surrounding the relationship between expectation and conditioning, and the extent to which each contributes to eliciting a placebo response. By the 1990s, Fabrizio Benedetti, a neurologist in Turin, began a series of mechanistic studies that launched us into the modern era. These would set the stage for two decades of placebo neuroimaging studies that were set in motion by landmark papers in pain, depression, and Parkinson's disease, and would transform the way we think about placebos today.[19]

Midway through, in 2010, Ted Kaptchuk and colleagues founded the Program in Placebo Studies (PiPS) at Harvard Medical School. This was the first multidisciplinary organization for placebo studies. Compared to previous placebo research, which was typically conducted by individual researchers in their area of expertise, PiPS assembled a team of clinicians, psychologists, anthropologists, philosophers, biologists, neuroscientists, and geneticists to conduct research that was translatable to the clinic. A few years later, in 2014, the Society for Interdisciplinary Placebo Studies (SIPS) was founded by some of the PiPS members and other leading international placebo researchers. SIPS is an international organization that promotes communication and collaboration between research centers and scholars in the study of placebos, use of multidisciplinary tools to investigate the psychological and physiological mechanisms of the placebo effect, and translation of these findings into ethical methods to utilize placebo effects in the clinic.

In Regione Vivorum

Since Mesmer versus Franklin and Perkins versus Haygarth, we have done an outstanding job separating clinically effective treatments from those that appear to have no benefit beyond that of a placebo. But like Franklin, Haygarth, and the many scientists and clinicians who followed, we have failed to focus on the most important part of the placebo puzzle: the patient. While the determination of safety is paramount and immutable, the determination of efficacy presents a different challenge. If both a placebo and verum pill, injection, or surgery equally reduce patient suffering with no difference in benefit, is it fair and reasonable to withhold both when there is no other option available?

It has taken hundreds of people performing thousands of experiments with tens of thousands of patients to bring us to this moment (figure 4). In the chapters that

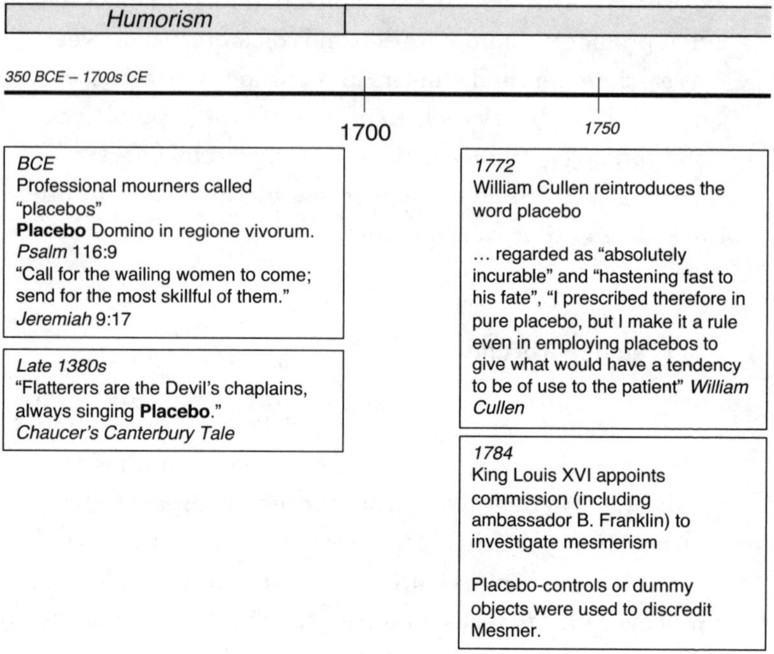
Humorism
350 BCE – 1700s CE
1700
1750
BCE
Professional mourners called "placebos"
Placebo Domino in regione vivorum.
Psalm 116:9
"Call for the wailing women to come; send for the most skillful of them."
Jeremiah 9:17
Late 1380s
"Flatterers are the Devil's chaplains, always singing **Placebo**."
Chaucer's Canterbury Tale
1772
William Cullen reintroduces the word placebo
… regarded as "absolutely incurable" and "hastening fast to his fate", "I prescribed therefore in pure placebo, but I make it a rule even in employing placebos to give what would have a tendency to be of use to the patient" *William Cullen*
1784
King Louis XVI appoints commission (including ambassador B. Franklin) to investigate mesmerism
Placebo-controls or dummy objects were used to discredit Mesmer.

Figure 4 The timeline of research areas, medical approaches, and major events in the history of placebo effects.

Patent Medicine

1800   *1850*   Civil War   1900

1800
Haygarth investigates Perkins' tractors

1807
Jefferson comments on placebo

"One of the most successful physicians … assured me, that he used more bread pills, drops of colored water, & powders of hickory ashes, than of all other medicines put together. It was certainly a pious fraud…"

1897
Pavlov observes classical conditioning

1905
AMA starts "Seal of Acceptance" program for advertisement in AMA publication, JAMA

1903
Richard Cabot comments on placebo
"[I was] brought up, as I suppose every physician is, to use placebo, bread pills, water subcutaneously, and other devices . . . I doubt if there is a physician in this room who has not used them and used them pretty often . . . I used to give them by the bushels"

Figure 4 (continued)

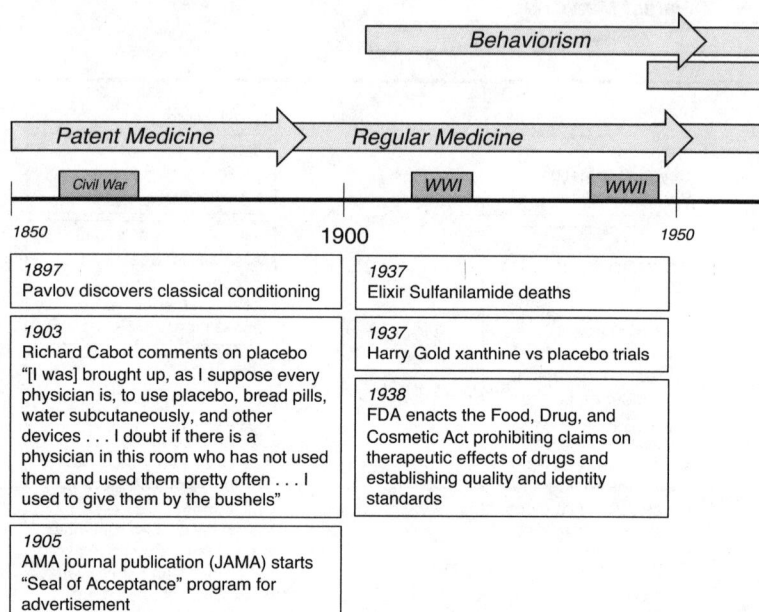

Figure 4 (continued)

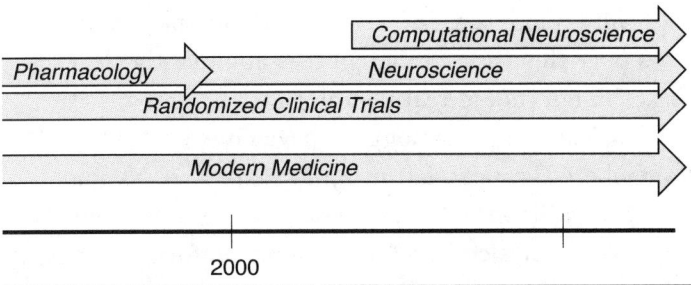

1955 Henry Beecher reviews randomized controlled trials and identifies placebo effect "It is evident that placebos have a real therapeutic effect being produced in 35% of cases." (below)	*Early 2000s* Seminal neuroimaging papers fundamentally shift understanding of the placebo mechanism *Wager et al., 2004 (below)* *Petrovic et al., 2002* *Mayberg et al., 2002* *De la Fuente-Fernandez et al., 2002*
1975 Ader and Cohen condition an immune response in rats	*2008* Kaptchuk et al. demonstrate multiple treatment non-specific factors contribute to the placebo effect
1978 Levine et al. demonstrate that naloxone extinguishes placebo effect	*2009, 2011* Eippert, Bingel et al. demonstrate the role of endogenous opioids in placebo effect using PET; show that placebo effect can downregulate pain stimulation in the dorsal horn of the spinal cord.
1985 Kirsch introduces concept of response expectancy, and suggests expectancy and classical conditioning underlie placebo response	*2010* Kaptchuk et al. performs open-label placebo study in IBS patients
1992 Buske-Kirschbaum et al. conditioned an immune response in humans	

Figure 4 (continued)

follow, I will explore some of what we have learned about placebos over this time. Although it is abundantly clear that placebo effects are real neurological responses that elicit changes in our physiology, we have not traveled too far from where Haygarth left us on January 1, 1800. Placebo research still bears the stigma of quackery and deceit, making many a physician and scientist uncomfortable. In many respects, in the land of the living, placebos are still in mourning.

HOW EXPECTATIONS AND CONDITIONING SHAPE PLACEBO EFFECTS

It was time for Dr. Musavi to convey the sad news. With her health rapidly declining, his patient, Mrs. Ozra, had less than two weeks to live. Summoning the family together, he encouraged them to make arrangements. Although it was obvious to the clinician, this news came as a surprise to the family. Ozra's oldest son, Arman, had been living in exile for the last twenty years, and it would be hard for him to return to say goodbye. They begged the doctor to do all he could to extend her life until they could get Arman home. Musavi paused for a moment, "There is a new treatment that I could try," he said, "It's been having some promising results. I could try it on your mother." With hope and relief, the family gave Musavi permission to proceed.

It took over a month for the family to get Arman home. By the time they brought him to his mother, the transformation was evident. Ozra had a surprising return to health. When she passed over a year later, the family contacted Musavi to thank him for the lifesaving treatment. "Can I tell you a secret?" he asked, in a hushed tone, "It was only sugar cubes."[1]

What if what you expect to experience from a treatment influenced how well the treatment works? If this were true, then past experiences, observations of the experience of others, and verbal suggestions could also influence your symptoms. And what if you were unaware that the treatment was inert, that it was a placebo? Would your experience of the treatment's effects be more like the treatment you think you are getting or like a placebo?

There is considerable experimental evidence that expectations drive our experience of treatment regardless of whether the treatment is a drug or placebo. When the treatment is inert, the experience of benefit is called a placebo effect. A popular model of how placebo effects work proposes that expectations lead to psychophysiological effects, which in turn reduce symptoms. In addition to expectation, placebo effects can be shaped by associative learning. Associative learning or conditioning is the process by which a symbol (i.e., a bell or pill) is repeatedly paired with a stimulus (i.e., food or pain reduction), and as a result, the symbol or cue alone elicits the effect of the original stimulus. Conditioning and expectation are not separate processes but rather represent a continuum by which information is processed and used consciously or unconsciously by an individual to guide perception and response. In this chapter, I will examine how conditioning and expectation influence placebo effects.

Associative Learning from Mice to Men

Classical conditioning, the process of training or habituating a human or animal to respond to a stimulus in a certain way, derives from the methodology laid out by the Russian physiologist Ivan Petrovich Pavlov in the early 1900s. Pavlov repeatedly paired the sight and smell of food, which naturally causes dogs to salivate, with an unrelated neutral but novel event like the ringing of a bell.[2] After a number of repeated pairings, the ringing of the bell alone induced salivation independently of the presence of the sight or smell of food. Although the connection of Pavlov's finding to placebo effects is patently clear in hindsight, it would take another half century before we made the leap to conditioning drugs in humans.

In 1962, Richard J. Herrnstein (who would coauthor the controversial *The Bell Curve* thirty years later) reported the conditioning of placebo effects in rats.[3] By repeatedly pairing saline injections with scopolamine, a drug that depresses muscular movement and coordination,

Herrnstein was able to depress movement in the rodents by saline injection alone. In subsequent conditioning experiments, other researchers demonstrated that animals could be conditioned with other drugs like morphine or amphetamine. But not every drug had the expected effect. In 1971, Robert Pihl and Jack Altman paired saline with the tranquilizer Thorazine. Instead of conditioning depressed activity, the rats were more active than ever with the subsequent saline injections.[4] Pihl and Altman reasoned that there is likely an interaction between the nature of the drug being studied and the response being measured. Thorazine inhibits dopamine signaling in the region of the brain involved with learning.[5] Could Thorazine be an exception to the conditioning paradigm because it blocked the acquisition stage of learning? Could Thorazine be one of those drugs like naloxone that can perturb a placebo response? I will return to the question of when and how drugs like naloxone disrupt a placebo response in chapter 3.

While exceptions to the conditioning paradigm remained a curiosity, studies rapidly progressed to conditioning the immune function. As with many important discoveries in science, the finding that immunosuppression could be conditioned in animals occurred by chance. Taste aversion studies in rodents date back to the 1940s. The British Army, trying to eradicate rodents from foxholes during World War II, observed that rats would sparingly sample a poisoned food and then assiduously avoid subsequent exposures to it. Rats are unable to vomit to purge themselves of toxic substances, and hence taste aversion is an important adaptation that helps them avoid drinking or eating potentially noxious substances. Taste aversion is rapid and persists for over a month, and thus provided researchers with an excellent animal model for studying associative learning with other drugs like lithium chloride, morphine, and cyclophosphamide. Early studies pairing saccharin with cyclophosphamide, an immunosuppressant drug, found that many of the conditioned animals died when they were rechallenged with saccharin.[6] Interestingly, the rate at which they died was correlated with the amount of saccharin they consumed. As it was well known that saccharin did not kill rodents, these findings suggested that the conditioning protocol caused an overactive immunosuppressant response to the saccharin, which in turn led to the demise of the animals. In 1975, Robert Ader and Nicholas Cohen followed up on these initial findings, and demonstrated that indeed pairing a drinking solution of saccharin with an injection of the immunosuppressant cyclophosphamide could induce immunosuppression when the animals subsequently drank saccharin alone.[7] This study inspired a series of experiments in which specific immune function changes, like the reduction in white blood cell count, weight reduction in the spleen and thymus, and changes in cytokines, could all be conditioned by varying the specific immunosuppressive drug. The inverse was also true. Enhanced immune function could be conditioned by pairing saccharin with drugs that activate white blood cells.

Immune modulation in animals was soon translated to humans.[8] In 1992, Angelika Buske-Kirschbaum and colleagues paired sherbet with an epinephrine injection, which is known to elicit an increase in natural killer cell activity. When given sherbet with a saline injection, the conditioned group showed an increase in natural killer cell activity.[9] In subsequent years, the conditioning of placebo effects became an established protocol.[10] Today, researchers are actively exploring using conditioning, or as it is currently termed, associative learning, to reduce the use of opioids. In these "dose-extension" studies, placebo pills are interspersed with verum opioids, and through associative learning, the dose of pain treatments can be gradually reduced and replaced with a placebo.[11]

Although compelling as the mechanism by which placebos mediate their effects, classical conditioning falls short of explaining key features of placebo effects. In the clinical setting, the response to a placebo can be induced by less deliberate processes than conditioning. Further, potent pharmacological drug effects can be modified by suggestion. For instance, the pain-killing effects of morphine are substantially reduced when its administration is hidden from the patient.

For a while there was a robust debate regarding the difference between conditioning and expectancy.[12] This debate, however, resolved with the understanding that both expectation and conditioning require some level of association between the "inert" (e.g., a placebo pill) and "active" (e.g., a drug) stimulus that requires cognitive processing. After all, Pavlov had to pair the smell and sight of food with the bell, or he could ring the bell till the cows came home and nobody would salivate.

Great Expectations

One of the most striking examples of how expectation can influence symptom relief is the mirror cure for phantom limb pain.[13] The amputation of an arm or leg can leave many patients still experiencing the limb as if it were present, and sometimes this causes extreme pain in the "phantom limb." In 1992, Vilayanur Ramachandran developed a simple and ingenious treatment. He placed patients beside a mirror box (figure 5) in which they could see their remaining limb reflected in the mirror. This gave the patients the impression that they were viewing their real and healthy original limb. While looking at the image of their hand in the mirror, the patients were instructed to send movement commands to both of their limbs and make symmetrical movements that one would typically make with

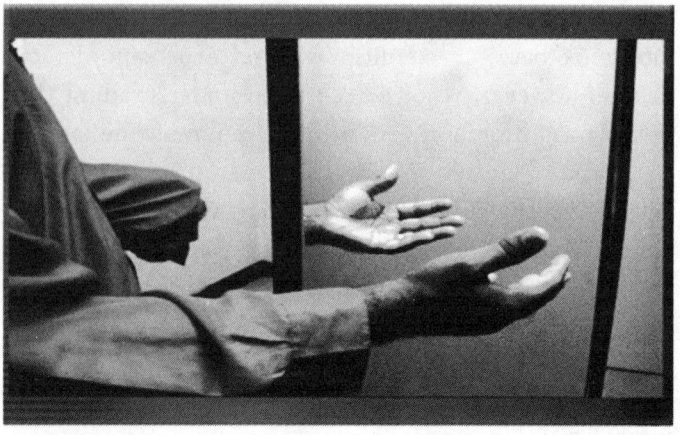

Figure 5 The mirror box for treating phantom limb pain. *Source*: V. S. Ramachandran and E. L. Altschuler, "The Use of Visual Feedback, in Particular Mirror Visual Feedback, in Restoring Brain Function," *Brain* 132, no. 7 (July 2009): 1693–1710, https://doi.org/10.1093/brain/awp135.

both limbs. In the case of an amputated hand, they could make the motions of conducting a band, or opening and closing both hands. Quite miraculously, as they watched "both their hands" seemingly functioning normally, they experienced an amelioration of the pain. Thus mirror visual feedback (MVF), as this procedure is called, builds an experience of their phantom hand as functional, pain free, and able to enact commands that shift the expectation of how their hands feel. MVF, which is remarkably effective at ameliorating phantom limb pain, is by no means inert and is not formally considered a placebo treatment, but

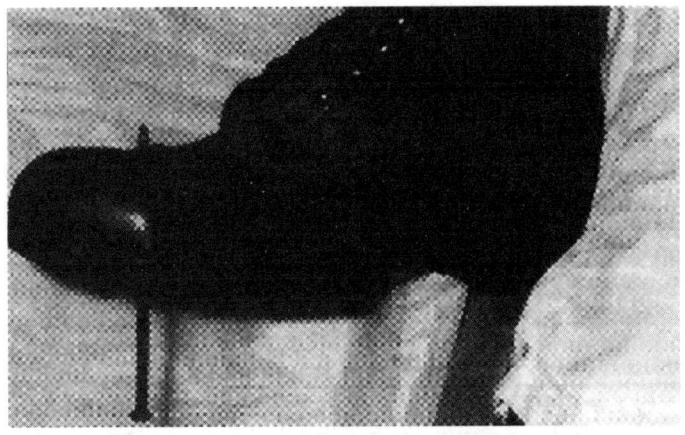

Figure 6 Image of the boot of twenty-nine-year-old construction worker who accidentally landed on a seven-inch nail that went right through his boot. He was admitted to the hospital in severe pain. When the boot was removed, it was revealed that the nail passed between his toes not through his foot.

this therapy underscores the power of our perceptions in having a hand in modulating our symptoms.

Expectations can relieve as well as induce pain. In 1995, a twenty-nine-year-old builder was rushed to the emergency department at Leicester Royal Infirmary after jumping down onto a seven-inch nail that went right through his boot.[14] He was sedated with midazolam and fentanyl as the slightest movement of the nail was extremely painful (figure 6). After carefully removing the boot, it was immediately apparent that while the nail had entered proximal to the steel toe cap, it had slid between the builder's toes, and his foot was entirely unharmed. This information immediately relieved the man's pain.

In a Word

The term *expectancy* is common in the placebo literature and refers to the unconscious predictions that individuals hold.[15] Just as Ozra expected benefit from Musavi's treatment, and the builder expected pain from the seven-inch nail in his boot, expectations in the context of a placebo (response expectancy) is theorized to elicit the suggested or believed response because the subject expects it to do so.[16] Expectations are shaped by learning from past experience, informed by contextual verbal and nonverbal cues, and can be either positive or negative. Thus through placebo mechanisms, expectations can enhance or minimize the effects of a treatment.

The effects of expectation on pharmacologically active treatments was elegantly demonstrated in a study in which Ulrike Bingel and colleagues used three different conditions with verbal instructions to manipulate the effects of the powerful painkiller remifentanil.[17] Remifentanil is a fast-acting opioid analgesic administered by infusion and used to manage pain after surgery. In this experimental setting, healthy individuals were hooked up

Expectations are shaped by past experience, and can be either positive or negative. Through placebo mechanisms, expectations can enhance or minimize the effects of a treatment.

to an infusion pump, and asked to rate a painful thermal stimulus that was administered before and during the infusion at various time points. Throughout the experiment, the information given to the participants about the infusion was changed to modulate expectancy, but the level of the thermal heat pain stimulus remained the same across the whole experiment. At the baseline when the saline infusion was initiated, the participants were asked to rate their pain on a scale of zero to a hundred. The average pain rating at the baseline was sixty-six. Without the awareness of the participants, the remifentanil infusion pump was then turned on and ran for the duration of the experiment. After thirty minutes of "hidden" remifentanil infusion, the second thermal pain stimulus was administered. Again the participants were asked to rate their pain. This time, they rated their pain slightly lower, at around fifty-five, suggesting only a small benefit from this potent drug. The investigator then told the participants that the infusion was about to begin, even though it had already started. With this "open" remifentanil infusion, a positive expectancy was created. When, once again, the same pain stimulus was administered, the participants rated their pain to be much lower, at around thirty-nine. Hence there was significantly less pain experienced with "open" compared to "hidden" remifentanil. Finally, the participants were told that the infusion was being stopped and they might expect an increase in pain with the next thermal stimulus. Although the infusion was not stopped, when once again they got the same pain stimulus, as a result of negative expectancy, they now rated their pain significantly higher, at about sixty-four. The pain rating with this second "hidden" remifentanil condition was almost back to the baseline level before the remifentanil infusion was initiated. The researchers also measured unpleasantness and anxiety, and found similar results to the pain ratings. By concealing the identity of the infusions, Bingel and colleagues were able to isolate the effect of verbal information and visual cues on pain and unpleasantness ratings, and demonstrated that these cues modulate treatment outcomes significantly (figure 7). While positive expectancy dulled the participants' pain, negative expectancy actually exacerbated pain, in spite of the powerful analgesic.

The Bingel study was not the first to document the malleability of pharmacological effects; it was preceded by numerous studies that demonstrated that verbal suggestion could induce the opposite of the expected effects. For example, verbal suggestion could reverse the analgesic effects of nitrous oxide, elicit sedative effects with epinephrine, amphetamine, and aspirin, and induce stimulating effects with the sedative chloral hydrate.[18] Using the open-hidden paradigm, with informed consent, the effects of powerful drugs like diazepam were reduced by 50 percent if the administration was hidden.[19] Similarly, when the administration of the drugs buprenorphine, tramadol,

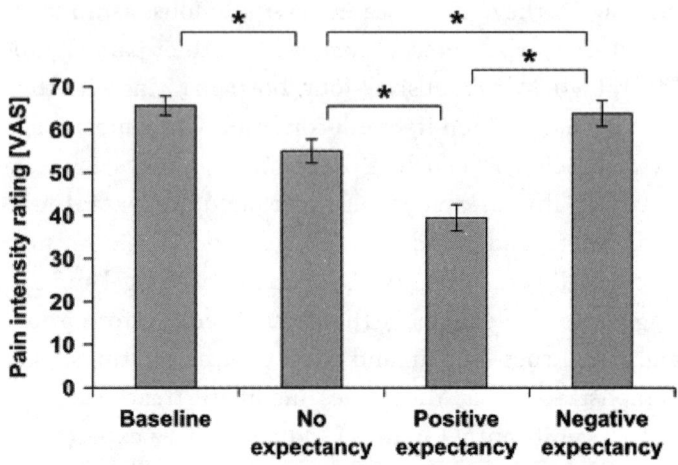

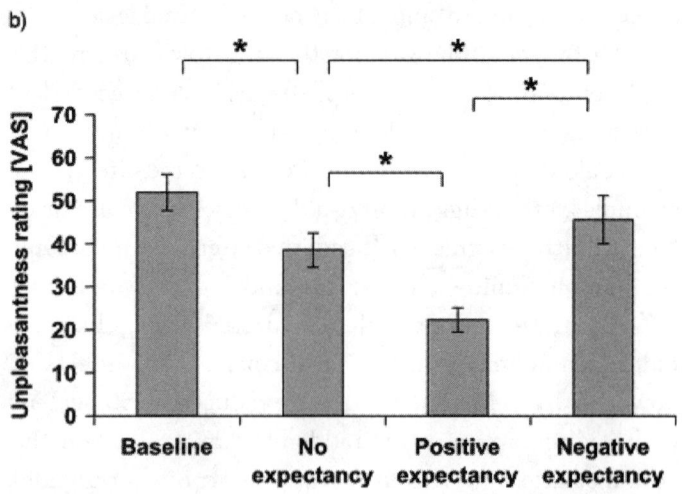

ketorolac, and metamizole was hidden, 50 percent more drug was needed to elicit the typical analgesic effects observed when these drugs were administered openly.[20]

The labeling of drugs can also have a strong influence on expectation and consequently treatment outcomes. A good example of this is the migraine study done by Slavenka Kam-Hansen and colleagues comparing the effects of labeling a placebo and Maxalt (the brand name of rizatriptan, an effective headache medicine that works by narrowing the blood vessels in the brain).[21] In the study, matching bottles containing a placebo or Maxalt were labeled as "placebo," "Maxalt," or "placebo or Maxalt." Thus the bottles were either correctly, incorrectly, or ambiguously labeled. The order in which the patients were supposed to use the pills from each of these bottles was randomized for each participant; for the next 6 migraine attacks, they would use pills from the bottles in the order that they were assigned. The patients were asked to report their level of pain thirty minutes after the onset of a headache (the baseline) and then take study pills from the designated bottle. Two and half hours after a headache onset, they were asked again to record their level of pain.

Figure 7 The behavioral effects of expectation modify opioid analgesia.
(a) Ratings of pain intensity on a visual analogue scale (zero to a hundred).
(b) Ratings of pain unpleasantness after each of the four experimental runs.
Notes: Error bars indicate SEM. *$P < 0.05$.

After 459 headaches, the results were in. Maxalt labeled as Maxalt was the most effective at treating the headaches, but there was no difference statistically between Maxalt mislabeled as a placebo and a placebo mislabeled as Maxalt (figure 8).

One Gets What One Pays For

The influence of expectations on treatment outcomes is not limited to explicit manipulations of information in the clinical encounter. Studies examining manipulations of cost, branding, and subtle cost-related cues have found that patients hold subconscious associations between cost, branding, and treatment efficacy that influence treatment outcomes. Study participants who receive a treatment that "costs more" tend to experience a greater benefit as compared to when they receive a treatment that "costs less," even when the treatments are identical and inert.[22] Even switching between brands, especially from a name-brand to a generic, has been shown to modify subjective and objective outcome measures of efficacy.[23]

Expectation-related effects can also be transmitted by social observational learning. Social observational learning occurs when the observation of a demonstrator's behavior modifies the behavior of the observer. When combined with other nonverbal cues, conditioned social

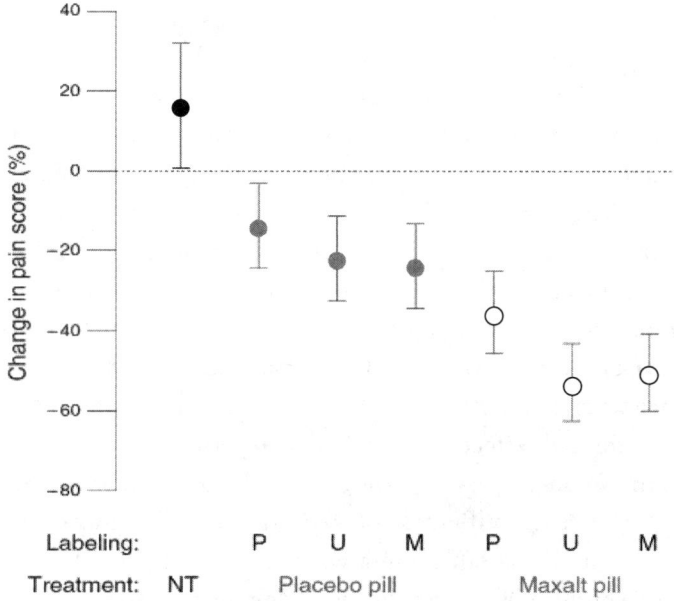

Figure 8 Changes in headache intensity in response to a placebo (gray dots) labeled as a placebo, unlabeled, or Maxalt, and Maxalt (white dots) labeled as a placebo, unlabeled, or Maxalt. The no treatment control (NT) is the black dot. This figure shows that there was no difference between Maxalt labeled as a placebo and a placebo labeled as Maxalt.

learning can enhance placebo responses.[24] This effect can cause negative responses too; a good example of this phenomenon in clinical trials is the increased likelihood of patients' experience of side effects after hearing about them from other patients, even if the patients are taking a placebo. These nocebo effects are somewhat common in clinical trials and will be discussed in chapter 4. In an influential study, patients were randomized to a placebo or montelukast, an active treatment for asthma, with neutral or positive treatment expectations. Strikingly, participants given literature that mentioned headaches as a possible side effect of montelukast experienced headaches more frequently, even if they were taking a placebo.[25]

Given the influence of expectations on clinical outcomes and side effects in a wide cross section of studies and conditions, more attention could be paid to the information that patients are exposed to during clinical trials. On the one hand, there is an ethical imperative in shared decision-making between the patient and clinician that calls for the patient to be fully informed about the potential benefits and risks involved in a study.[26] On the other hand, the very act of informing the patient about the benefits and risks of the study shapes the benefits and risks of the study. How to balance these competing ethical imperatives to provide what is truly of benefit to the patient remains in question.

While expectation was thought to be a behavioral response, in the last twenty years, neuroimaging studies have revealed the regions of the brain that are modulated by both positive and negative expectations. In the next chapter, I will take a look at these neurobiological mechanisms underlying the potential of expectations, and in turn placebos, to drive clinical effects.

THE BRAIN ON PLACEBOS

Perception of an object costs
Precise the Object's loss—
Perception in itself a Gain
Replying to its Price—

The Object Absolute—is nought—
Perception sets it fair
And then upbraids a Perfectness
That situates so far—

—Emily Dickinson, "Perception of an Object Costs," 1866

At the start of the new millennium, a series of ground-breaking neuroimaging studies moved placebo effects from the domain of behavior to the business of the brain. As we saw in the last chapter, expectations and associative learning powerfully influence placebo effects. But how do these behavioral influences coupled with an inert pill or sham intervention induce brain signaling to produce placebo effects?

The brain during pain is a particularly useful model for studying placebo effects because pain is easily manipulated in laboratory settings, and the neural process of nociception (the perception of pain from a noxious stimulus like heat or mechanical pressure) is experimentally reliable and well studied. Thus most placebo neuroscience research has focused on pain and placebo-induced pain relief or analgesia in healthy controls.

With elaborate ruses designed to manipulate expectations or induce associative learning, placebo neuroscientists have used neuroimaging to examine the brain before, during, and after a painful stimulus plus placebo treatment. Over the last two decades, these elegant and ingenious experiments linked distinct brain regions with responses to a placebo. The findings of these studies demonstrated that our brains form predictions of how an incoming stimulus will be experienced based on contextual cues, prior experiences, and expectations. These predictions are encoded in neurological activity driving mechanisms that override the information carried in incoming pain signals to shape our perception. So thermal heat at the same temperature can be experienced as more or less painful depending on what we think about the nature of the pain we are about to experience.

In this chapter, I will concentrate first on neuroimaging studies of placebo analgesia and a recent working model used to explain what is happening to the brain on placebo. I will then discuss changes in the brain related to placebo-induced symptom relief in conditions like Parkinson's disease or depression. Let's start with a little background.

The Brain in Pain

The human brain is a uniquely complex organ that on the surface, appears not to be doing a whole lot. On closer inspection, however, by recording from single nerve cells or using neuroimaging techniques like functional magnetic resonance imaging (fMRI) or positron emission tomography (PET), we see that the eighty-six billion nerves or neurons, neatly organized by function, are in constant communication. Therefore neuroimaging allows us to objectively examine the mechanisms involved in generating placebo effects.

Information moves within as well as between neurons by electric signaling and neurotransmitters. Neurotransmitters are small molecules or chemicals produced in the body that are passed from one neuron to the next, exciting or inhibiting downstream signaling by binding to proteins on the surface of neurons called *receptors*. The two main neurotransmitters implicated in placebo effects are opioids and dopamine. Opioids bind to opioid receptors and are involved in the transmission of pain relief signals. The mu-opioid receptor is the most widely studied type of opioid receptor, and is responsible for binding to endogenous (made in the body) opioids and painkillers like morphine. Dopamine binds to dopamine receptors, and is involved in signaling related to reward and physical movement. Though dopamine and opioids are the most commonly studied in placebos, other molecules that have effects in the brain, like the hormone vasopressin, have recently caught the interest of neurobiologists and been shown to have effects on placebo responsiveness.[1]

Damage to bodily tissues causes pain or nociception. This type of pain is sensed by specialized nerve cells or neurons called nociceptors. Nociceptors carry pain signals up from the peripheral regions of the body to the central nervous system, which consists of the spinal cord and brain. Pain signals that enter the spinal cord at the dorsal horn are routed up to the base of the brain or brain stem. From there they are directed to the "pain matrix," a group of brain regions involved in the emotional, cognitive, and motor aspects of pain experience.[2] The regions of the pain matrix are linked by neural circuits and include the *thalamus*, which relays motor and sensory pain signals; *hypothalamus*, a major control center connecting hormones to the nervous systems that regulates body temperature and blood pressure; *amygdala*, involved in emotional responses, particularly feelings of anxiety, fear, pleasure, and response to threat; *insula*, which mediates emotion, empathy, and interpersonal experience; *somato-sensory cortex*, which receives and processes pain; and the *anterior cingulate cortex* (ACC), involved in emotion, empathy, and decision-making. As we will soon see, regions of the pain matrix are also recruited in the processing of placebo-induced pain relief or analgesia.

Opioids and Pain

Pain is an almost universal human experience. Though it manifests uniquely in individuals, pain is one of the most common reasons patients seek medical attention. The most enduring and popular of pain treatments comes to us from the poppy plant, which contains opium, a highly addictive pain-relieving narcotic. The opiates morphine, codeine, and heroin are derived from the resin of the poppy seed capsule. While opiates are naturally occurring, the endogenous opioids enkephalin and endorphin are made in the human brain, and opioids like OxyContin, hydrocodone, fentanyl, and remifentanil are synthetic. Like opiates and synthetic opioids, endogenous opioids modify pain signals by binding to opioid receptors, proteins located on the surface of neurons. Many of the brain regions associated with pain-signal processing have high concentrations of opioid receptors, making them natural targets for pain relievers and placebo effects.

Placebo Analgesia in Neuroimaging Studies

To carry out placebo studies in the laboratory setting, neuroscientists developed a working model of pain stimulus and placebo analgesia.[3] The general format of these studies starts with a scan of the brain to determine baseline activity. This is followed by a training phase in which a painful stimulus (e.g., thermal heat) is delivered to a readily accessible region on the body of the subject (e.g., the forearm) while they are in a neuroimaging scanner. The subject is asked to rate their pain on a visual analog scale from zero, the equivalent of "no pain," to a hundred, indicating the "highest imaginable pain" intensity. The brain is scanned to determine activity with pain exposure. In expectation experiments, the subject is then given a placebo cream or injection with verbal suggestions that create an expectation of benefit, or reduction in the experience of pain from the intervention. Unbeknownst to the subject, the painful stimulus is then reduced so the subject begins to think that the placebo is actually effective at reducing the experience of pain. This step is sometimes repeated to reinforce the association between the placebo intervention and reduction in pain. After this associative learning phase, there is a testing phase in which the subject is given the original level of pain along with the now deemed "effective" placebo intervention. The brain is scanned several times throughout the experiment to determine differences in brain activity with and without expectation of protection from the painful stimulus. The difference between the level of pain experienced before and after the placebo intervention is considered a measure of the placebo effect.

In the over three hundred placebo neuroimaging studies, there have been numerous iterations of the experimental model of pain and placebo analgesia. There have been variations in types of pain (e.g., pressure, heat, or electric shock), instructions (e.g., positive or negative), and conditioning cues (e.g., syringe, cream, or pill). Some studies use associative learning with a powerful painkiller like morphine or remifentanil to maximize the placebo effects or a drug that blocks opioid signaling like naloxone to block the placebo effects. Today, neuroimaging studies coupled with increasingly sophisticated and powerful computational models are revealing the inner workings of the brain during placebo analgesia.

Brain Activity during Placebo Analgesia

Placebo neuroscientists are able to take advantage of the binding of neurotransmitters to their receptors by using radioactively labeled versions of neurotransmitters to track the receptor-binding activity as a proxy for receptor activity. Radioactive carfentanil is a radiopharmaceutical that is molecularly similar to the synthetic opioid fentanyl and can be detected using PET.[4] In PET brain imaging, subjects are infused with a radiopharmaceutical that emits gamma rays detected by gamma cameras to create a three-dimensional image of the brain. After over twenty years of neuroimaging studies using PET and other modalities, the specific regions of the brain involved in placebo-induced analgesia have been revealed.[5]

An early clue that endogenous opioids were involved in placebo analgesia came from studies in the late 1970s that found that pretreatment with the drug naloxone could abolish placebo effects.[6] Naloxone is a drug that works by blocking opioid binding to mu-opioid receptors and is used today under the trade name Narcan to reverse opioid overdoses. The finding that naloxone can also reverse placebo responses has been replicated numerous times. We now know that placebo effects induced by both expectation and conditioning with the opioid morphine can be at least partially blocked by naloxone.[7]

In one of the earliest neuroimaging studies, brain activation in response to a placebo was compared to that seen with remifentanil, an opioid with analgesic potency comparable to fentanyl.[8] In this study, thermal pain administered a few seconds before a PET scan reliably demonstrated increased activity in regions of the pain matrix, including the thalamus, insula, and ACC. Before the administration of subsequent painful stimuli, subjects were told they would receive an injection of one of two powerful painkillers. In actuality, the painkillers were remifentanil or placebo saline. Both remifentanil and the placebo effectively reduced the pain experienced by the subjects. Remifentanil and the placebo also induced similar increases in brain activity in the rostral anterior cingulate cortex (rACC, a subsection of the ACC that has a high density of opioid receptors and is activated with opioid treatment) and periaqueductal gray (PAG, an area in the brain stem that plays a role in motivated behavior and response to threatening stimuli, and is important in descending pain modulation). The observation that the activation of the rACC covaried with the activation of PAG provided early evidence that placebo effects could lead to the interception of incoming pain signals and exert "top-down" control over the pain. In top-down processing, our brain's expectations and prior knowledge reinterpret or change the perception of an incoming sensory signal. Put simply, placebos allow our brains to experience sensory signals for pain as less painful.

Further placebo analgesia experiments revealed that the coactivation of the rACC and PAG was correlated with multiple other factors: it was proportional to the magnitude of the placebo response, correlated with reduced signaling in the pain matrix somatosensory cortex, could be blocked by naloxone, and was associated with reductions in activity in the rostral ventromedial medulla (RVM), a key structure located in the spinal cord that is also involved in the top-down pain modulation system.[9]

The Very Major Placebo Frontal Commander

Tor Wager is among the placebo neuroscientists who have generated substantial evidence that the ventromedial prefrontal cortex (vmPFC), located proximal to the rACC, is a key region in integrating memory, prior experience, context, expectations, and incoming sensory information to generate placebo effects. As a main change center, it appears that the vmPFC uses this integration of information to override sensory inputs, changing the way we think about our surroundings and experiences. In this top-down manner, the vmPFC redirects our interpretation of the moment. Thus it is not surprising that the vmPFC, or what I call the "very major placebo frontal commander," has emerged as a central region of interest in placebo research (figure 9).

One way to invoke top-down pain modulation is through cognitive reappraisal. An example of using cognitive reappraisal in medical settings is encouraging subjects or patients to think about a painful stimulus or symptomatic pain as a "warm blanket on a cold day" rather than as

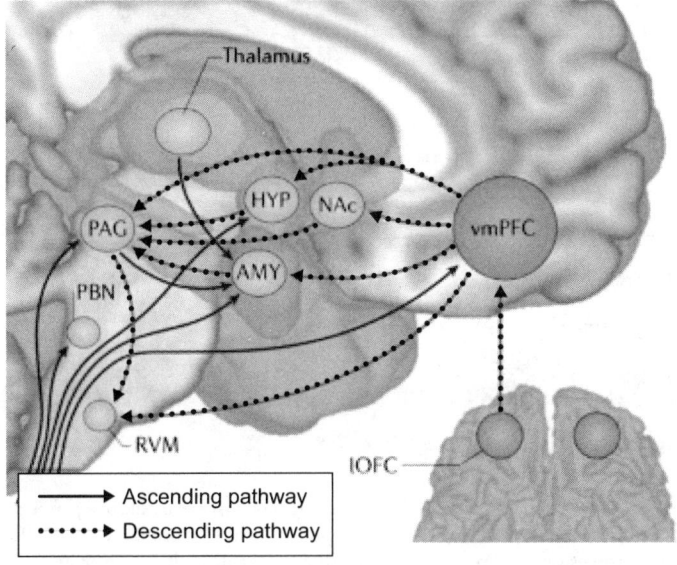

Figure 9a Converging ascending and descending pathways. NAc is nucleus accumbens, HYP is hypothalamus, AMY is amygdala, PAG is periacqueductal gray, RVM is rostral ventral medulla, PBN is parabrachial nucleus, and lOFC is lateral orbitofrontal cortex, part of the prefrontal cortex. *Source*: T. D. Wager and L. Y. Atlas, "The Neuroscience of Placebo Effects: Connecting Context, Learning and Health," *Nature Reviews Neuroscience* 16, no. 7 (July 2015): 403–418, https://doi.org/10.1038/nrn3976.

b)

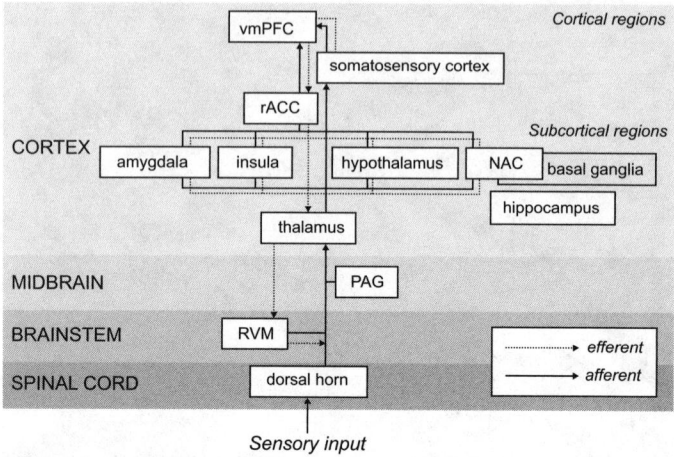

Figure 9b   A simplified map of the brain regions active in a putative placebo effect network. In pain, incoming nociceptive signals (red lines) ascend to pain-processing brain regions that include the amygdala, thalamus, insula, and somatosenory cortex. The top-down modulation of the incoming pain signals is influenced by the vmPFC and rACC cortex, which project to pain-processing centers, which in turn project to PAG, RVM, and ultimately the dorsal horn of the spinal cord.

a sharp pain. In trials of cognitive reappraisal across disease models, the vmPFC is consistently activated. Further, the vmPFC is associated with the control of emotional responses, self-control, and decision-making, and is highly connected to the rest of the brain.[10] Increasing supportive care and touch are two factors of the therapeutic relationship demonstrated to activate the vmPFC.[11] Interestingly, structural differences in the vmPFC have been observed in multiple conditions known to have a high placebo response in clinical trials, including depression, attention deficit hyperactivity, substance misuse or addiction, schizophrenia, and dementia.[12] Outside psychiatric challenges, the vmPFC has been shown to be activated during meaning-related tasks like the formation of therapeutic relationships.

Top-Down Processing and Placebo Effects

In top-down processing, perception is driven by cognition; we leverage what we already know or have experienced to build a model or expectation that shapes what we experience. To get a better sense of how top-down processing works, take a look at the two boxes below.

We read the context of the top box as a sequence of letters and might perceive the middle character to be the letter B in the sequence A, B, and C. In the lower box, we see a sequence of numbers and read the same character in the first box, now displayed in the middle of a string of numbers, as the number 13.

12 13 14

What does top-down processing have to do with placebo effects? As we will see in the upcoming sections, behavioral and neuroimaging experiments provide compelling evidence that placebo analgesia is a special case of a top-down modulation of pain signals. This evidence dates back to work done by Howard Fields in the 1960s in which he demonstrated that analgesia could be induced by direct electrophysiological stimulation of the PAG. The PAG is the same region in the brain stem that years later was found to have increased opioid signaling in concert with the rACC during placebo-induced pain relief.[13] Fields proposed that incoming pain signals traveling up through the spinal cord could be perturbed in a top-down fashion. More recent neuroimaging studies showed that this top-down pain modulation could, like placebo analgesia, be blocked by naloxone. To examine how top-down modulation works, placebo neuroscientists like Christian Buchel turned to a framework or model called predictive coding.

Predictive Coding toward a Model of Precision and Placebo Analgesia

It is intriguing to consider where Emily Dickinson (1830–1886) in her "Perception of an Object Costs" derived the inspiration for what arguably is the most succinct and elegant explanation of predictive coding. Perhaps it was through her close relationship with the mathematician Susan Gilbert that Dickinson learned of the theories of Hermann von Helmholtz (1821–1894). Helmholtz was a German physician and physicist who in the 1860s argued that our perceptions were not a direct projection of the world around us but rather a constructed model of the world based on a succession of learned "unconscious inferences."[14]

More recently, British neuroscientist Karl Friston, building on Helmholtz's theory, proposed that our brains are prediction machines. Friston contends that in order to keep us safe and able to operate efficiently in a noisy, stimulus-filled world, we cut down on background noise and focus in on the most important stimuli in a given instant.[15] To be able to do this, our brains construct models of what we will experience in the upcoming moment. Instead of waiting to take in and process all available information, we predict our experiences—what we will see and how we will feel—sometimes before we are fully aware that there is something to see or feel. In so doing, we constrain our perceptions and reactions to what we expect will happen next. In concentrating on only a subset of incoming information, we are more efficient with our finite energy resources.

As one of the most recent and compelling models of placebo analgesia, predictive coding benefits from the power of neuroimaging to capture the timing and magnitude of brain activity in response to stimuli that vary in intensity, and thus vary in precision. Placebo neuroimaging studies designed to test the validity of using a predictive coding model in placebo analgesia not only support predictive coding as a model that explains how placebo effects work but also demonstrated that the precision or surety of our expectations can have a profound influence on the nature of our experience.

The model holds that the expectations induced by associative learning and/or placebo treatment recruit top-down opioid-mediated signaling at key regions in the spinal cord, limiting incoming signals to the pain matrix. In so doing, a patient's experience of pain can be reduced by their expectations. Hence the precision of a subject's expectation can be manipulated by repeatedly exposing them to variable pain levels during the associative learning phase of an experiment.[16] For instance, subjects who get consistently lowered heat stimuli with the administration of a placebo cream have a more precise expectation and consequently more robust placebo response. In

We predict our experiences—what we will see and how we will feel—sometimes before we are fully aware that there is something to see or feel.

contrast, subjects exposed to greater variability in heat stimuli levels during the associative learning phase of the experiment have a weaker placebo response. This study therefore supported the hypothesis that both the expectation and incoming stimulus are weighted by their relative precisions to shape the experience of pain and placebo effects. Dickinson, ahead of Helmholtz and Friston, alludes to this transactional nature of precision in the relationship between "the object absolute" and how we situate or "set it fair" with our perception: "Precise the Object's loss— / Perception in itself a Gain / Replying to its Price."

Other Conditions and Models

While pain is a convenient model to study placebos, placebo analgesia studies are limited by being mostly performed in healthy volunteers. Understanding the neurological mechanisms in conditions that are characterized by high placebo response rates in clinical trials, like Parkinson's disease and major depression, is critical to being able to identify and evaluate effective treatments for these illnesses.

Parkinson's is a neurodegenerative disease characterized by reduced motor function with tremors, slowness, and general difficulty controlling movement. A common neuropathic anomaly in patients with Parkinson's disease is a loss of dopamine-signaling neurons specialized in instructing and implementing motor functions. The placebo effects in Parkinson's disease are high but variable, ranging from 0 to 55 percent, and can result in tangible long-term improvements in motor function.[17]

In a seminal study on placebo effects in Parkinson's disease, the placebo treatment induced the release of endogenous dopamine in the areas of the brain responsible for planning movement, learning, reward, motivation, memory, emotion, and action.[18] Not surprisingly, the magnitude of the dopamine release was greater in the patients who reported a placebo benefit compared to those who did not. These findings, replicated in numerous subsequent studies, point to dopamine and dopamine signaling in the striatum (a brain region involved in decision-making and movement) as another important neurological region involved in the production of placebo effects.[19] In placebo studies in patients with Parkinson's, it appears that the expectation of receiving a reward (a benefit from the drug), not the reward itself, is linked to increased dopamine release in the ventral striatum. Recordings from individual neurons revealed that the response to a placebo was associated with changes in the basal ganglia circuit, a region implicated in Parkinson's disease.

Major depression is another condition characterized by a high placebo response in clinical trials.[20] Studying the antidepressant effects of placebos is difficult because of the typical delay in responses to pharmaceutical treatment, which tend to occur across weeks to months rather than within minutes to hours. Still, several studies have made important contributions to our understanding of placebo-induced neurological mechanisms in depression. In an early placebo antidepressant imaging study, patients with depression were scanned using PET before and after a six-week treatment with the antidepressant fluoxetine (Prozac) or a placebo.[21] In this pivotal study, placebo and fluoxetine responders showed overlapping neural activity in several brain regions, suggesting common pathways shared by placebo and antidepressant treatments.

Since this early study, there has been extensive research to assess the placebo response in individuals with depression, particularly because the rates of a placebo response in patients with depression continue to be quite high, stumping the development of novel antidepressants. Recent PET studies found that antidepressant placebo effects in patients with depression increased brain activity through the transmission of both dopamine and opioid neurotransmitters.[22] These results support theories that the opioid and dopaminergic pathways are involved in placebo responses, though they might have separate and compounding effects.

The Brain and Placebos

Pain, Parkinson's disease, and depression are models that show significant changes in the brain in response to placebo treatments, allowing for the dissection of mechanisms underlying placebo effects in healthy controls and patients, but they are not the only ones that show neurobiological changes. Additional placebo effect models are being developed in other conditions, including irritable bowel syndrome (IBS), asthma, and Alzheimer's disease. These models suggest that there are multiple disease-specific and common pathways engaged in the formation of placebo effects. Importantly, an expectation of benefit plays a critical role in the magnitude of the alleviation of the perceived symptoms and response to placebo treatment across disease models. Expectations are significant, and the mechanism that placebo recruits is powerful. The vmPFC has emerged as a key region in using our expectations to shape placebo effects. Thus we might consider the vmPFC to be a *back door* to how we see and experience the world—a back door that is susceptible to being hijacked by manipulative messaging. While underlying placebo effect mechanisms can be used for good, negative information and expectations can have the opposite and sometimes negative effects. This phenomenon, termed the nocebo effect, is where I begin in the next chapter.

NOCEBO EFFECTS IN MODERN MEDICINE

Very superstitious,
Writing's on the wall,
Very superstitious,
Ladders 'bout to fall,
Thirteen month old baby,
Broke the lookin' glass
Seven years of bad luck,
The good things in your past
When you believe in things
That you don't understand,
Then you suffer,
Superstition ain't the way

—Stevie Wonder, "Superstition," 1972

Superstition, in particular negative superstition, is the most common form of nocebo in everyday culture. From breaking a mirror, to walking under a ladder or stepping on a crack, superstition attributes cause of a consequent action or event to logically unrelated preceding actions or events. This misattribution is characteristic of how nocebos, and in turn expectations, can shape perceptions and the meanings we make of the experience of subsequent exposures. In the extreme, there is documented evidence that fears from strongly held cultural beliefs can induce the ultimate nocebo effect: death. A team of researchers found that Chinese Americans who believe in Chinese astrology, and "have a combination of disease and birth year which Chinese astrology and medicine considers ill-fated," die younger than patients with the same disease that were born in a different year. According to the researchers, the "strength of commitment to traditional Chinese culture" correlated with the difference in life span. This surprising phenomenon is evident in several other cultures where the power of a hex or curse can invoke cultural beliefs resulting in unexplained sickness, sleep paralysis, and even sudden death.[1] Though you might take these extreme nocebo examples with a grain of salt, you probably have not been above tossing a pinch of salt over your shoulder from time to time.

As we saw in previous chapters, positive expectations can induce neurological changes that enhance the effectiveness of a treatment and lead to the production of placebo effects and amelioration of symptoms. Unfortunately, the inverse is also true. Negative verbal suggestion, associative learning, and contextual cues create negative expectations that are accompanied by neurological changes that can increase the experience of symptoms. This phenomenon, termed the nocebo effect, is the antithesis of the placebo effect. Derived from the Latin *nocere*, "to harm," Walter Kennedy coined the term *nocebo* in 1961 to describe the impact that negative suggestions or information can have on clinical outcomes. In this chapter, I examine the neurological circuitry activated by nocebos, and discuss the factors that promote the negative expectation and transmission of nocebo effects in randomized clinical trials, popular culture, and the clinical encounter. Strategies to mitigate nocebo effects will also be explored.

The Brain on Nocebo

Not surprisingly, there are similarities between the neurological pathways that mediate placebo and nocebo effects. The expectation of a negative experience (i.e., pain) creates a mental representation of the pending experience by activating the prefrontal cortex (PFC), ACC, and vmPFC. The thalamus and insula, two regions that encode pain, are activated too. When an individual is exposed to the painful stimulus, their experience is proportional to the combined effect of the intensity of the stimulus and precision of the expectation. If the expectation is for less pain, more often than not, less pain is experienced. If the expectation is for more pain, the experience of pain is frequently amplified.[2] The worker landing on a seven-inch nail in chapter 2 is a perfect example; observing the nail through his boot, he anticipated and felt extreme pain, even though the nail wasn't penetrating his foot at all. In this way, negative expectations drive nocebo-induced hyperalgesia or increases in pain.

Nocebo-induced hyperalgesia can be observed through brain imaging in real time. Pain and the expectation of pain induces activation in overlapping brain structures. These structures include the regions of the pain matrix discussed in the earlier chapters along with the thalamus, insula, dorsolateral prefrontal cortex, ACC, and somatosensory cortex. Whereas positive expectations dial down signaling in pain-related regions, negative expectations can enhance this signaling. Nocebo effects are not limited to placebo studies in hyperalgesia; nocebos and their harmful effects are everywhere. To get a sense of real-world nocebo effects, let's take a look at statins, side effects, and cardiovascular disease.

Statins and Cardiovascular Disease

As a young man, Akira Endo was inspired by Alexander Fleming and the discovery of penicillin. After college in

Nocebo effects are not limited to placebo studies in hyperalgesia; nocebos and their harmful effects are everywhere.

Japan, he spent two years in New York City, where he was struck by how many people suffered from cardiovascular disease, the leading cause of death in the United States. Cholesterol was in large part to blame. Endo reasoned that if mold made molecules that killed bacteria, perhaps they also made molecules that could perturb cholesterol synthesis. On returning to Japan, he screened culture broths from thousands of mold extracts in search of an anticholesterol "antibiotic."

It was the 1970s, and Endo was about to revolutionize cardiovascular disease prevention. Compactin, the molecule he discovered, had potent lipid-lowering effects in animal models, but in his clinical trials in patients with severe familial hypercholesterolemia, an inherited form of high cholesterol, one of the subjects experienced muscular dystrophy. Although this side effect disappeared when the treatment was stopped, it was enough to halt development of compactin. Luckily, Merck, a pharmaceutical company, took up the cause, and soon after another mold extract, lovastatin, gained regulatory approval. In all, seven statins including atorvastatin (Lipitor) and rosuvastatin (Crestor) would do well in clinical trials, and make it to the now-competitive statin market.

Statins are remarkably effective at lowering low-density lipoprotein or the "bad" cholesterol. Patients taking statins have almost a 50 percent lower risk of heart attack, stroke, or the need for bypass surgery.[3] Overall, statin users have a 20 percent lower chance of dying from any cause compared to their counterparts who don't take a statin. But despite this impressive efficacy, statins could never shake the stigma of muscle pain.

Statin Denialism and the Nocebo Effect

While statins *can* cause muscle pain, arguably most muscle pain and other statin-related adverse effects are not caused by the drug but instead by nocebo effects. To ensure patient autonomy and decision-making power, it is important to ensure that the patient is fully informed about possible negative outcomes of potential treatments. The informed consent procedure in randomized clinical trials requires the disclosure of all the possible side effects associated with a given treatment. Because statins do induce myopathy and rhabdomyolysis, or muscle wasting, in rare cases, this information has to be communicated to patients in clinical trials to allow them the autonomy to decide if the drug is right for them. Incredibly, the side effects observed in the *placebo* arm of a trial are strikingly similar to those explained and attributed to the active treatment in informed consent. Up to a quarter of the patients in the placebo arm of statin clinical trials drop out because they experience adverse effects.

Information about the potential side effects of statins is not limited to informed consent in clinical trials. It is not even limited to shared decision-making discussions in the clinical setting. Negative information about statins is everywhere. A recent Google search of "statin side effects" produced over ten million hits; many of these sites post unsubstantiated theories about why statins are harmful and cause harmful adverse effects. A common trope is that statins inhibit cholesterol, and as your brain is made of cholesterol, statin use can shrink your brain. As a result of what seems to be a campaign of misinformation, many who might benefit from taking a statin to reduce their risk of cardiovascular disease opt not to.

An N-of-1 Study

One of the many studies used to get to the bottom of the statin side effect conundrum was an n-of-1 clinical trial in which patients served as their own controls by taking either the statin or a placebo control for specified time intervals. Between 2016 and 2019, sixty patients who had previously discontinued statin use within two weeks of starting treatment due to side effect complaints were enrolled in the trial.[4] These patients each received a month's worth of atorvastatin, a placebo, or no pills for one-month intervals over a twelve-month period. The order in which they were instructed to take the pills varied between the patients and was randomized from month to month. The patients reported their daily symptom intensity on a scale of 0 (no symptoms) to 100 (worst symptoms) via a smartphone app. If their side effects were too strong, they could stop taking that set of pills for the rest of the month and resume with the next designated set of pills the following month.

At the end of the n-of-1 study, the researchers found that during the no-pill month, the average pain intensity was 8.0; during placebo months, it was 15.4; and during statin months it was 16.3. Therefore taking any pill increased average pain, but there was little statistical difference between the average statin and placebo-related pain intensities. Of the enrolled sixty participants, forty-nine completed the trial, and thirty were able to restart statin treatment without difficulty after the trial. This study not only supports the assertion that statin-related side effects are commonly misattributed to the drug but also underscores the ethical predicament facing clinicians: on the one hand, too little information robs the patient of their autonomy; on the other hand, too much negative information can induce nocebo effects, and lead to poor adherence to or rejection of a treatment that might be of great benefit to the patient.

Common Nocebo Effects Associated with Other Drugs

Statins are not the only drugs plagued by nocebo effects. The suggestibility of side effects is observed in many other conditions. Meta-analyses (a systematic assessment of the results of multiple clinical trials) of side effect suggestibility in patients being treated for migraines or using SSRIs found that the adverse events reported tended to be closely related to those of the active substance in the trials.[5] For example, erectile dysfunction (ED) is a commonly cited symptom of beta-blockers, a blood pressure medication.

In a study in which ninety-six male patients were randomized to a beta-blocker, subjects given no information about the treatment had few cases of ED (3.1 percent), those given the name of the treatment, "atenolol," reported more cases (15.6 percent), but almost a third of the patients who were given the name of the drug and information about side effects reported ED (31.2 percent).[6] In the second part of this study, those participants who reported experiencing ED were rerandomized to receive a placebo or Sildenafil, a drug that treats ED. In the study, the placebo and Sildenafil were equally effective at reversing ED. This trial clearly demonstrates the potency of negative as well as positive expectations to influence clinical outcomes. It is possible that anxiety about this particular side effect in the first part of the study contributed to a higher incidence of ED. This link between nocebos and anxiety is emblematic of the potential of negative experience and nocebo effects in the context of clinical care to lead to worse clinical outcomes. But this is just the tip of the iceberg of the pain and suffering that nocebo effects can cause.

Nocebo Effects in the Clinic

Studies have shown that when patients walk into a doctor's office and experience being seen and heard by a doctor who is present and attentive, their treatment outcomes are far more successful. Components of the treatment encounter, including therapeutic alliance, warmth, and competence, have been shown to augment treatment outcomes. In one of the landmark papers in the placebo literature, participants with IBS were randomized to three groups that re-created an increasing "dosage" of the clinical encounter. The minimal dose was just an assessment or observation of symptoms. Adding the ritual of treatment by a clinician to the observation had a stronger effect. Establishing a positive relationship between the patient and treatment practitioner during treatment by ensuring eye contact, listening to the patient's symptoms, expressing confidence in the treatment, and emphasizing physical touch was the strongest dose of placebo.[7] One can imagine that the absence of these placebo-enhancing elements in the clinical encounter could reduce the quality of the treatment. In other words, the absence of placebo-inducing effects could result in suboptimal care.

With the ethical challenges of creating negative experiences, less has been done to modify and study negative physician encounters. Lauren Howe and colleagues, however, used an allergic reaction paradigm to study practitioner effects.[8] In this study, an allergen was administered in a pinprick, followed by a topical inert cream, and then either positive ("that the cream would reduce the reaction and itching") or negative ("that the cream would increase the reaction and itching") information was provided by a clinician who demonstrated either high or low warmth and competence. The size of the wheals among the participants who were randomized to the positive framing was significantly smaller than among those given the negative framing. Surprisingly, regardless of expectation, the participants randomized to the high warmth, high competence clinician interaction had the smallest wheal size. In this way, the impact of expectations on allergic reactions was enhanced when the clinician demonstrated warmth and competence, and this effect was nullified by a cold and less competent physician.

Nocebo and Racism in the Clinical Encounter

Although not commonly framed in nocebogenic terms, implicit bias and racism can seed negative expectations and drive nocebo effects.[9] Just as important, the absence of placebogenic factors can also lead to negative clinical outcomes. Substantial evidence suggests that nonwhite patients often receive unfavorable treatment in comparison to their white counterparts.[10] This disparate, frequently inferior treatment is characterized by less empathy and time spent with patients, poor communication, and less caring behavior on the part of physicians.[11] Other studies found that physicians were less likely to participate in shared medical decision-making or establish rapport with nonwhite patients, and that nonwhite patients were less likely to receive sufficient information.[12] In another study, independent, nonbiased raters found that physicians were 23 percent more verbally dominant and 33 percent less engaged in patient-centered communication in medical visits with Black patients as compared to white ones.[13]

Given the potential for nocebos to cause harmful effects, it is important that clinicians and physicians understand their mechanisms of action, and what steps can be taken to mitigate their effects.[14] Generally, experts agree it is important to educate physicians and patients about the potential for nocebo effects in a way that matches the clinical context.[15] These experts and other clinician placebo researchers encourage clinicians to help patients explore their concerns and expectations, and learn coping strategies to manage their expectations.[16] They suggest contextualizing worrisome information by setting patients' expectations of the information they will encounter on the internet and describing treatments in a realistic but positive way (i.e., present the proportion of patients who don't get side effects as opposed to the proportion who do get them).

In the specific encounter between white doctors and Indigenous, Black, or other people of color patients, antiracism training and communication and/or cross-cultural training to enhance clinician skills in caring for patients of other cultures or races is recommended to address the potential for the nocebo effects of racism and bias to negatively impact patient care.[17]

Nocebos in Popular Culture

Excipients are literally the stuff of placebos; they are the nonactive ingredients that allow manufacturers to compound a drug into a comestible pill with a reasonable shelf life. When Merck changed the excipients in the thyroid hormone replacement drug Levothyroxine from mannitol plus citric acid to lactose, it set off a virtual firestorm. Before releasing the new formulation, Merck had conducted a randomized bioequivalence study that found that the biological outcome measures were essentially identical and the new formulation was completely safe. Nonetheless, patients reported significant side effects; from hair loss, headaches, and weight gain, to diarrhea, extreme fatigue, and increased heart rates, the rash of side effects experienced by the tens of thousands of patients with hypothyroidism in France gave rise to more than sixty lawsuits accusing Merck and the French government of a "failure to assist a person in danger."[18] Finally, the minister of solidarity and health asked Merck to bring back the old formulation, and the outcry died down. At the same time, the company introduced the new formulation in other countries, with more deliberate communications to patients about the change.

A similar mass nocebo effect happened a decade earlier in New Zealand. In 2007, GlaxoSmithKline moved the manufacturing of Eltroxin, the only thyroid hormone replacement drug approved for use by the New Zealand government, from Canada to Germany, resulting in some changes to the inert components of the drug's formulation. Though the new manufacturing process was actually more expensive than the old one, some New Zealanders believed that the switch was a cost-cutting tactic of the pharmaceutical company that put patients at increased risk. A local pharmacist was concerned about the adverse events he observed in patients and reported them to the media. The story of a "small town health professional taking on the 'medical establishment'" gained widespread media attention, and an almost two thousandfold increase in reported adverse events followed.[19] Conspiracy theories proliferated that the company was lying to patients and that the new formula contained genetically modified or toxic agents. Studies at the time showed that the regions with the most media coverage of the switch also tended to have the highest rates of reported adverse events. Some of the adverse events reported were consistent with hypothyroidism, but a great number were nonspecific. After testing, it was determined that the new and old drugs were bioequivalent, and once it was announced that an alternative drug would be made available, the adverse events dwindled significantly. Clearly, nocebo effects transmitted through media can be pervasive, and have widespread public health impacts that severely affect treatment outcomes and adherence.

In the midst of the COVID-19 pandemic, nocebos and their effects are increasingly relevant. Opportunities for nocebo effects to influence behavior and outcomes are rampant.[20] Combined with potential preexisting medical mistrust, the stress of deciphering misinformation or conspiracy theories, and the dramatization or exaggeration of potential virus symptoms and vaccine side effects in the media, the scene is set for nocebos to take over. Though it is difficult at this time to assess how many of the COVID-19 vaccine-related side effects, which include headache, fatigue, fever, and sore arms, are potentially influenced by nocebo effects, a recent initial meta-analysis found that there is a high rate of adverse events reported in patients assigned placebo shots.[21] Though at this point it would be hard to prove, the impact of media hype about these side effects likely has the downstream effect of creating vaccine hesitancy. While people need to be informed about the potential risks of the vaccine, broadcasting those risks does indeed appear to be exacerbating the nocebo effect.

In the United States, fear and misinformation about the vaccine side effects are prevalent and surveys in 2020 showed that a substantial portion of people were unsure about the COVID-19 vaccine or did not plan to get the vaccine when it became available to them.[22] Consequently perhaps, the rates of vaccination are relatively low; the Mayo Clinic reports that in the United States as of 2021, only 67 percent of the eligible population has received a first dose, and an average of about a thousand people die a day from the virus.[23] Portugal, on the other hand, boasts one of the highest vaccination rates in the world; with 86 percent of its total population fully vaccinated, and 98 percent of the eligible population fully vaccinated, Portugal was able to lift all COVID restrictions and had a death rate of less than ten per day in 2021.[24] As we all know, the COVID-19 landscape is changing rapidly, and it remains to be seen if nocebo or placebo effects will prevail.

PLACEBOS IN CLINICAL TRIALS

> After thousands of studies, hundreds of millions
> of prescriptions and tens of billions of dollars in
> sales, two things are certain about pills that treat
> depression: Antidepressants like Prozac, Paxil and
> Zoloft work. And so do sugar pills.
> —Shenkar Vedantam, *Washington Post*, 2002

There are many potholes on the long road from "bench" laboratory discovery to "bedside," the clinical setting in which drugs are prescribed to patients. After discovering a protein or pathway that impacts a particular disease, drug developers spend years honing small synthetic or large biological molecules that target and they hope will perturb the disease process. A lead molecule is chosen based on its selectivity for the target, and then preclinical scientists characterize the molecule's metabolism, excretion, and safety in animal models. Only after clearing these hurdles is the molecule ready for testing in humans via the phases of clinical trials. In small phase I trials of twenty to eighty healthy volunteers, the safety and dose are determined. If that goes well, the next step is testing for the efficacy in increasingly larger phase II (one to three hundred patients) and then phase III (one to three thousand patients) placebo-controlled clinical trials. If patients give their informed consent to join the study, they are randomized to either the study drug or placebo control arm of the trial.

Placebos as Controls in Clinical Trials

Placebos in clinical trials are used to control for regression to the mean, Hawthorne effects, the natural history of the condition, and of course, placebo effects. Regression to the mean in clinical trials is a statistical phenomenon in which particularly high or low measurements or readings, when repeated at a later date, will tend toward the average. This is important in clinical trials because patients have a tendency to enroll in trials when their symptoms are at their worst and therefore can appear to have improved regardless of the intervention.

The Hawthorne effect is named for a series of commissioned lighting studies conducted at the Western Electric factory near Chicago between 1924 and 1927. The studies were designed to determine whether workers were more efficient in bright or dim lighting. During the study, worker productivity was enhanced with all illumination intensities, but returned to prestudy levels once the study was completed. After several other similar experiments, it was determined that it was the observation and monitoring of the workers that was driving improvements in productivity. Thus the simple act of enrolling in a clinical trial, completing questionnaires about the state of one's condition, and being observed by a clinician can influence and in some cases ameliorate symptoms.

Natural history refers to natural symptom fluctuations expected in the course of a condition. A good example of this is the common cold. If a researcher conducted a two-week study on the common cold, it is quite likely everyone would respond to treatment at the end of the study not because the treatment worked but rather because colds generally get better in about a week.

Finally, placebo effects, the subject of this book, are physiological responses to the therapeutic context and treatment delivery that can themselves result in clinical improvements sans active intervention. There is a general bias or expectation on the part of clinicians as well as patients to believe that patients who receive the active treatment are more likely to get better. Hence to avoid bias and the influence of expectations that can enhance placebo effects, studies are "double-blinded" so that neither the patients nor the clinicians know whether the patient is receiving the active study drug or an inert placebo.

To receive FDA approval, drugs tested in "pivotal" phase II and III trials must produce a significantly greater clinical benefit compared to a placebo control. Failure to beat the placebo response is one of the most common reasons why drugs "fail" in clinical trials of neurological and psychological conditions.[1] There is a high price to pay for these failures. A 2020 study from the London School of Economics estimated the median cost of bringing a new drug to market at \$985 million, with an average cost of \$1.3 billion.[2]

When drugs fail, the reverberations across patients' lives can be widespread, and impact prognosis, quality of life, and emotional well-being. Furthermore, when these novel treatments, many with compelling mechanisms of action, are shelved, companies can fail, and jobs are often lost. The fault, of course, is not with placebos; many drugs just don't work. A survey of phase III trials in 2016 indicated that most fail because of a lack of efficacy, and a majority of these trials were in oncology, a field in which demonstrating a survival benefit in patients with cancer is a critical and high bar.[3] In neurological (e.g., Alzheimer's disease), psychiatric (e.g., depression), and functional pain (e.g., IBS) illnesses, however, the response to the placebo treatment is commonplace and can tip the balance in failure's favor.

Placebo Controls in Alzheimer's Trials

It has been almost twenty years since the FDA approved a new drug for Alzheimer's disease, a progressively debilitating neurodegenerative condition resulting in brain changes that can severely impair cognition. It is a late onset condition characterized by memory loss, confusion, mood changes, difficulty understanding and processing information, and general cognitive decline. In 2019, Alzheimer's was the sixth leading cause of death in the United States. In 2021, 1 in 9 people over the age of sixty-five and a total of 6.2 million people in the United States were diagnosed with Alzheimer's disease.[4] Today, there is no cure. As our population ages, the prevalence of Alzheimer's is increasing, along with its enormous attendant social and economic burdens.

Although deficits in expectation-mediated placebo responses have been observed in patients with Alzheimer's in an experimental setting, robust placebo responses in clinical trials have thwarted even the most promising drug development programs.[5] To tackle this problem, nonprofit organizations like TransCelerate and the Critical Path Institute are leading efforts to harness the collective knowledge in historical placebo controls to model disease progression, and understand when and how randomized drug and placebo treatments can influence this progression.[6] Such efforts call for generosity and trust among drug manufacturers as they pool their resources, successes, and failures to tackle the many obstacles in getting much-needed drugs to patients.

Drugs designed to prevent disease progression and treat Alzheimer's target the many interrelated pathologies that result in some of the biological correlates of the disease, including protein aggregation, amplified oxidative stress, neuroinflammation, and impaired neurotransmission in the brain. The deposition of amyloid-β (Aβ) plaques and neurofibrillary tangles are characteristic findings in the brains of patients with Alzheimer's. One approach to preventing the neurodegeneration and neurotoxicity associated with Aβ plaques is to use antibodies, large biomolecules naturally generated by the body, to bind to and clear out this unwanted material.

Biogen in Cambridge, Massachusetts, is a US biotech company that developed one of the first promising monoclonal antibody therapies, aducanumab, that targets Aβ plaques.[7] In preclinical mouse studies, Biogen demonstrated that aducanumab entered the brain and reduced plaque formation in a dose-dependent manner. The Biogen researchers then moved on to small pilot studies in humans and had exceedingly promising results. After a year of monthly intravenous infusions, patients with mild Alzheimer's had reductions in brain Aβ plaques accompanied by a decrease in the rate of clinical decline. Importantly, the drug appeared to be safe and tolerable, albeit difficult to administer by infusion. Buoyed by these positive results, Biogen initiated two essentially simultaneous phase III clinical trials, a strategy to shorten the time to FDA approval.

Unfortunately, when the FDA independent advisory panel met at the end of 2020, it concluded that even the most compelling data did not support efficacy and voted overwhelmingly against approval. At issue were dose-dependent improvements observed with aducanumab that only separated from the placebo at the highest doses. Aducanumab, though seemingly safe, overall did not beat the placebo. Still, with no new drugs since 2003, Alzheimer's patient advocates and some patients who participated in the trial strongly encouraged the FDA to consider approving aducanumab. To the surprise of many, the drug was approved in 2021, and in 2022 the Centers for Medicare & Medicaid Services announced that Medicare would cover the new drug, pending further evidence of efficacy. With the contention around these developments, Biogen reduced the price of the drug by fifty percent in response to slow sales. Meanwhile, the failures of other Alzheimer's drugs continue to pile up; atuzaginstat from San Francisco–based Cortexyme, because of toxicity, and others like troriluzole from Biohaven Pharmaceuticals, based in Connecticut, were not approved because they failed to beat the placebo.

Placebo Controls in Clinical Trials of Depression

Alzheimer's disease is not the only therapeutic area battling placebo responses in clinical trials. Major depression is a chronic, recurring, and often debilitating psychiatric mood illness characterized by persistent feelings of sadness and anhedonia. In 2018, 264 million people worldwide were estimated to be affected by depression. The high prevalence of this condition comes at a growing cost. Since the introduction of fluoxetine (Prozac) to the market in the late 1980s, several other SSRIs have been approved by the FDA including sertraline (Zoloft) and paroxetine (Paxil). When asked, 75 percent of depressed patients said that they would prefer psychotherapy over antidepressant medication.[8] Nevertheless, with the demands on psychiatrists to treat the growing number of people suffering from depression, the expediency of prescribing a pill can frequently supersede the patient's preference for psychotherapy sessions. In 2019, the global antidepressants market was estimated at \$14.3 billion. The market surged to \$28.6 billion in 2020 as a result of the COVID-19 pandemic and is expected to level out at \$19 billion in 2023. Over the last twenty years, as Prozac, Zoloft, and Paxil became household names, a vigorous debate over whether they were any better than placebos played out among academic researchers and the press.

The first salvo in the antidepressant-placebo debate was fired in 1998 by Irving Kirsch, who was then at the University of Connecticut. Kirsch and colleague Guy Sapirstein published a controversial meta-analysis examining the average size of antidepressant effects compared to placebos in nineteen double-blind randomized clinical trials.[9] A meta-analysis is a statistical approach that allows researchers to combine results across clinical trials to get a sense of the overall effect of an "exposure," which in this case was antidepressants. Kirsch and Sapirstein found that the difference between the drug and placebos was vanishingly small. Based on the data, they estimated that placebos accounted for approximately 75 percent of the improvement ascribed to antidepressants. The remaining 25 percent could be attributed to an enhanced placebo response resulting from drug-induced side effects that allowed patients in clinical trials to "break-the-blind" and correctly guess that they were in the active drug treatment arm. As discussed in chapter 2, expectation is a critical driver of symptom improvement with placebo treatment; thinking that one is in the active treatment arm can lead to the self-fulfilling expectation of symptom improvement.

Four years later, in 2002, another meta-analysis, this time led by Arif Khan at Duke University, examined forty-five phase II and III antidepressant clinical trials in the

FDA database.[10] The FDA requires sponsors of clinical trials to submit their results regardless of whether the trials were positive (favoring the drug) or negative (favoring the placebo). This protocol is important to avoid publishing bias such that studies that are positive are more likely to be published in academic journals and thus more accessible to researchers than negative studies. While these data offered a more comprehensive look at the differences between antidepressants and placebos, this particular FDA data set only contained averages and did not include an estimate of the variability (i.e., no standard deviations or standard errors) so only simple data tabulations were possible. Nonetheless, Khan and colleagues found that the placebo response was a function of depression severity; in other words, the placebo response was smallest and the antidepressants were most effective among patients with severe depression.

Why were the antidepressant effects so small, and which patients were benefiting? By 2008, no fewer than 120 meta-analyses were published trying to identify the demographic variables (e.g., age and sex), comorbidities (e.g., bulimia), risk factors (e.g., smoking), and trial designs (e.g., placebo run-ins) that influenced the benefit from antidepressants. For the most part, the findings remained the same: little to no differences between the drug and placebo for mild depression, and significant but still relatively small benefit with an increased severity of depression.

In 2008, Kirsch, then at the University of Hull, invoked the Freedom of Information Act to access more comprehensive data submitted to the FDA.[11] Unlike the previous FDA data set, these data contained means and estimates of the variability. Still, the researchers found just small differences between the antidepressant and placebo. In that same year, Erick Turner at Oregon Health and Science University also published a meta-analysis combining published data with FDA data.[12] Turner found striking differences between the sizes of the effects reported in the published literature and the data available from the FDA. Almost all the antidepressant trials were positive in the published literature, but an analysis of the FDA data showed that only half of the registered trials were positive.

As Turner pointed out, this trend of the selective reporting of positive clinical trial results could have adverse consequences for researchers, patients, and health care professionals. Turner's meta-analysis found a small but statistically significant standardized mean difference (SMD) of 0.31 between the drug and placebo across all the data combined. The SMD is a summary statistic that makes it easy to compare the average effects across different outcome measures that might use different scales and different units. It is simply the difference between the average effect in the antidepressant groups minus the average effect in the placebo groups divided by the variability (standard deviation) among all the participants. In the published data, the result of the meta-analysis was higher: 0.41. Remarkably, both Kirsch and Turner found essentially the same SMD between antidepressants and placebos. Kirsch's SMD was 0.32.

With such similar results across these meta-analyses, one might wonder what was left to debate. It was the interpretation of the significance of these findings that was contentious. Turner, consistent with the data, argued that each drug was superior to a placebo. Kirsch, consistent with the National Institute for Health and Care Excellence (NICE) guidelines, contended that this incremental change was not clinically significant. In the United Kingdom, NICE provides national guidance and advice to improve health and social care. Early in the debate, NICE recommended that a three-point reduction in the Hamilton depression rating scale (HDRS) or SMD of 0.5 was to be considered clinically significant. In depression, clinicians frequently use the HDRS, a seventeen-item survey, to measure disease severity. This clinician-administered depression assessment scale asks patients about their feelings of sadness, guilt, anxiety, and sleep patterns. The higher the score, the greater the severity, and reductions in the score after treatment indicate improvement. Whether depression is mild, moderate, or severe is determined by the HDRS score at the beginning of the study. Thus Turner and Kirsch both had valid points. The question was, How much improvement in the HDRS should be considered clinically significant?

In 2018, the then largest of these dueling meta-analyses was published.[13] This time, researchers had the benefit of a recently developed, more powerful network meta-analysis tool; with twenty-one antidepressants in 522 trials comprising of 116,477 participants, they finally had "big data." Led by Andrea Cipriani at Oxford University, this impressive effort was as robust and rigorous as the preceding studies, if not more so, and once again the researchers found the same small but significant benefit of antidepressants over a placebo. Soon after, at the 2018 American Society of Clinical Psychopharmacology Annual Conference, Marc Stone of the FDA reported results from another analysis, arguably the most comprehensive.[14] This group from the FDA used all published and unpublished antidepressant trials sent to the FDA between 1979 and 2016. Like in the reports before him, Stone found the same small difference between the antidepressant drug and placebo response. With mounting criticism about the arbitrariness of its designation of clinical significance, NICE removed its recommended thresholds. Whether that small difference is clinically significant remains up for debate.

Minimizing Placebo Responses in Trials

Despite the consistent significant but small benefit of antidepressants over a placebo, the road to approval is still littered with near misses and failures, and some FDA decisions are still hanging in the balance. The failure to beat a placebo has been attributed to a myriad of factors: lax inclusion and exclusion criteria, the trial duration being too short or too long, a lack of adherence to the study drug, the wrong dose or formulation, the wrong study population, too small or too large trial sizes with too many sites, or the drug just doesn't work.

As many reasons as there are for failure, there are strategies in place to remove their influence. We can group these into three buckets: patient variables, clinical trial designs, and outcome measures. Ironically, with marginal differences between a drug and placebo, clinical trialists need to boost the statistical power by enrolling more patients into the trials. This need for more subjects has contributed to the globalization of clinical trials, which in turn has led to increased heterogeneity due to differences in access to clinical care (in some countries, enrolling in a trial is a way to get treatment), risk factors, and beliefs about health care that can influence expectations.[15] Trialists yielding to financial and temporal pressures might relax inclusion criteria, further increasing heterogeneity in the target population. Another problem is the growing cohort of professional patients who game the system by simulating patient effects to get enrolled in trials for money.

Adherence is also a critical factor in response to treatment. While medication adherence is likely a proxy for healthy behaviors, several studies have found that both drug and placebo adherence are associated with better health outcomes.[16] Still, poor adherence can in many cases be blamed for drugs failing to beat the placebo response. To address this problem, smart pill bottles are being deployed in clinical trials to monitor when patients take their study meds.[17]

Perhaps the biggest variable driving patient heterogeneity is the patient. In the case of depression, there is tremendous heterogeneity in the presentation and origin of symptoms. Some patients exhibit every symptom, and others only exhibit one or two. Some patients display depressive symptoms later in life after major events, and others show symptoms from a young age with no obvious "event." Because of these differences, it can be difficult to identify the mechanistic treatment needs of each individual patient based on the responses of the group. Add in gender, education, and social, psychological, and financial stressors, and you can see how the appropriate treatment could vary within just one individual at different stages in life, let alone for millions on a nationwide scale over time.

The elements of clinical trial design including the size, duration, number of treatment arms, and follow-up frequency are just a few of the variables that can influence outcomes in both the drug treatment and placebo arm of a trial. After more than seventy years of using placebo controls in clinical trials, we are only now starting to use historical placebo control data to map and project disease trajectories as well as predict placebo effects over time. Clinical trial designs that deviate from the gold standard of randomized placebo controls to managing placebo responses have had mixed results.

One such design, the placebo run-in, in which all the participants are given a placebo for the initial part of the study and then randomized, seemed like a great idea to weed out placebo responders. But this approach does not seem to lead to a greater effect size of the drug compared to a placebo.[18] Some sponsors initiate multiple phase II or III trials simultaneously at different doses, gambling that at least one or two of them will work, and thus they would have saved time. As in the case of the Alzheimer's aducanumab studies, this approach also has its drawbacks and can lead to confusion. More sophisticated trial designs are currently being investigated. One in particular, the sequential parallel comparison design (SPCD), has gained the recent attention of investors, media, and patients.

SPCD was designed by Maurizio Fava and David Schoenfeld at Massachusetts General Hospital in Boston with the aim of minimizing the effects of placebo responders. At first glance, the algorithm seems convoluted, but it makes a lot of sense. First, patients are randomized to a drug or placebo. After a prespecified period of time, those who don't respond to the placebo are rerandomized to a drug or placebo, but the placebo responders are kept on the placebo. The patients on drug in stage 1 stay on the drug throughout the trial. All the participants initially randomized to the drug stay on the drug. This innovative method was used most recently in the clinical trials of Alkermes's depression drug ALKS-5461 (pharmaceutical companies often affectionately name their drugs by their stock symbol plus a number). After two clinical trials, ALKS-5461, a fixed-dose combination of buprenorphine (a potent mu-opioid agonist) and samidorphan (a mu-opioid antagonist), failed to get approval from the FDA. While you might think the problem was that ALKS-5461 is an opioid seeking approval for treating depression in the throes of an opioid epidemic and COVID-19 pandemic, the impasse with the FDA appears to be related to disagreement over the use and analysis of the SPCD design. Ever cautious, the FDA is requiring more data from other trials to legitimize SPCD as an acceptable trial design. Quite naturally, drug sponsors are reluctant to run SPCD trials to produce the data without the assurance that the SPCD trials will be considered valid by the FDA. Given the importance of getting it right and the risks associated with being an early adapter, the future of novel designs will no doubt take some time to unfold.

Placebos in Clinical Trials: Where We Stand

The streptomycin and paluridine trials of the late 1940s are commonly touted as the first placebo-controlled clinical trials of the modern era, but they were preceded by the well-controlled patulin trial of 1944.[19] There was great promise that patulin, an antibiotic that like penicillin, was extracted from mold, was indeed the cure for the common cold. On Halloween 1943, the *Sunday Express* (London) heralded that "extensive tests—some on naval men—have since been carried out and it is believed they confirm its efficiency. The results of these tests are about to be published by the Medical Research Council."[20] But within months the disappointment and amnesia set in. The study conducted did not discern a difference between the drug and placebo.

Our ability to set aside disappointing results and move on to the next study is a hallmark of the resilience of drug discovery. Over the seventy-five years since these early trials, we have tended to rationalize and marginalize failures, while creating a story and vision of success for the next novel drug with compelling mechanisms of action, promising early efficacy and safety. Sometimes we get it right. In 2023, Merck's Keytruda, an antibody used in cancer immunotherapy, will become the best-selling drug in the world, projected to reach $22.5 billion by 2025. Yet increasingly in clinical trials of neurological and psychiatric

Through averaging, they completely miss the subset of people who have strong positive or negative responses to both the drug and placebo.

conditions, the number failing to demonstrate efficacy beyond the placebo control is growing.

Still, there is much hope. It is important to remember that the current analyses of trials look at the average effects across large groups of people. Through averaging, they completely miss the subset of people who have strong positive or negative responses to both the drug and placebo. While it is easy to do a post hoc analysis and say that older participants or patients with a certain genotype are likely to be placebo or drug responders, these subset analyses are frowned on. And for good reason, since the more specific subgroups you look at, the more likely you are to find a significant result just by chance. Further, original studies are carefully designed to have sufficient power to discern a significant effect. In subset analyses, the smaller sample sizes increase the likelihood of a false positive finding. Hence the holy grail in precision trials is to be able to predict who will respond or benefit from a therapy or even placebo.

As I will discuss in chapter 7, machine learning allows us to grapple with the complexity and heterogeneity in order to identify important patient- and clinical trial–level variables that enhance our precision. Patient-level variables include disease severity, age, sex, history of the condition, comorbidities, previous and current medications, neuroimaging data, and genomics. So it is here, amid the hills of heterogeneity, that the next great clinical trial challenge, precision trials and precision prescription, has set up camp.

THE PLACEBO EFFECT IN SURGERY

> The situation prevailing before, during, and after surgery is one usually filled with grave anxiety and stress. It would be surprising if, in this charged atmosphere, surgery did not have a powerful placebo action, in addition to what it may or may not accomplish physiologically.
>
> —Henry Beecher, "Surgery as Placebo," 1961

As a tennis and soccer player, I've had my share of, dare I say, successful surgeries. Over the years, I've peered at images of my torn ACL, meniscus, and rotator cuff, and listened carefully to surgeons explaining their plan of action. While the post-op pain was excruciating, especially for the rotator cuff, which involved the removal of bone spurs, I trusted my surgeons along with the generous use of ice, drugs, and physical therapy to get me back to the courts and pitch. And they did. So I must admit that I was one of the skeptics who found the results of the Can Shoulder Arthroscopy Work? (CSAW) clinical trial hard to believe.

CSAW, a randomized placebo-controlled clinical trial of subacromial shoulder impingement, compared the arthroscopic removal of bone spurs to sham surgery (arthroscopy only) or no treatment. Conducted in the United Kingdom, CSAW was a large multisite trial at thirty-two hospitals including fifty-one surgeons and three hundred patients with shoulder pain who were eligible for the surgery. This was a large study, so if there was a clinical benefit of the surgery over a placebo, this study had the statistical power to show it. Quite surprisingly, CSAW found that arthroscopic shoulder decompression, a hugely popular surgery, was no better than the placebo. Perhaps I should not have been surprised since this was not the first or even last time a popular surgery failed to demonstrate efficacy beyond that of a sham control.

Mammary Artery Ligation: An Early Casualty of Sham Surgery Controls

Four months earlier, a severe heart attack had left him a jobless semi-invalid. His breathing was labored, and his almost constant chest pain became severe on the slightest exertion. Two days after surgery he was out of bed, walking around his room. Pain had magically vanished; his breathing was improved. On the fifth day he went home and shortly thereafter he resumed work.

—J. D. Ratcliff, "New Surgery for Ailing Hearts," 1957

You might think that surgery and surgical procedures are the one medical intervention immune to the challenge of the placebo effect, but you would be mistaken. This epigraph is from a *Reader's Digest* story that boosted the popularity of a surgery called mammary artery ligation. The article chronicled the remarkable recovery of a sixty-one-year-old carpenter who received the surgery in Italy. In the early 1950s, angina pectoris (severe chest pain) was routinely treated by the bilateral ligation of the internal mammary artery, which is the internal thoracic artery that supplies blood to the chest wall and breast. This effective procedure was thought to work by increasing blood flow to the heart by collateral circulation.

While the surgery was widely viewed as successful in humans, in dogs it was a bust.[1] This failure to replicate the benefits of the surgery in an animal model inspired a 1959 double-blinded clinical trial to compare the ligation to sham surgery. The trial was carried out with seventeen patients, and outcome measures were obtained three to fifteen months postsurgery. All the patients were operated on, but only eight of them had verum ligation. Amazingly, during the first six months, about half the patients in each group (five out of eight for the ligated, and five out of nine for the nonligated sham) reported improvement in their symptoms, and two patients who were not ligated showed improvement in exercise tolerance.[2]

A follow-up study in 1960 used a similar procedure, comparing ligation to sham surgery, and found that improvement was similar among the patients who underwent ligation and those who had just the skin incision.[3] With these epic failures, the treatment was abandoned. Later, Beecher compared previously published ligation clinical trials.[4] He organized the trials based on the biases of the investigators and noted that studies conducted by "enthusiasts" tended to find positive results for mammary artery ligation; in the words of one enthusiastic researcher, "Practically all of our patients have had complete relief of the anginal pain." In contrast, studies conducted by "sceptics" found that few patients had complete pain relief.[5]

Despite Beecher decrying as immoral and unethical the continuation of "casual or unplanned new surgical procedures—procedures which may encompass no more than a placebo effect—when these procedures are costly of time and money, and dangerous to health or life," the use of placebo controls in surgical trials would be slow to catch on.[6] Still, placebo-controlled surgical trials continued to trickle in. For example, there was the pacemaker trial for obstructive hypertrophic cardiomyopathy that found no significant difference in perceived symptoms between the verum and sham surgery groups.[7]

Around the same time as the pacemaker trial, a trial of fetal tissue transplants in patients with advanced Parkinson's disease caused an ethical maelstrom. Although patients had for decades already been openly receiving the intracerebral transplantations, the results were mixed. The trial, conducted between 1995 and 1999, was designed to demonstrate the superior benefits of the surgery by randomizing patients to receive surgical fetal brain implants or a sham equivalent of the surgical procedure.[8] But from the start, ethicists raised concerns about the integrity of the human body and how the subjects would be able provide informed consent without there being therapeutic misconception. Some ethicists made the case that analysis of the individual patient's pre- and postoperative condition compared to patients who received standard treatments would suffice. Despite the resistance, the trial proceeded, and patients in both the verum and sham groups were given anesthesia, had holes drilled into both sides of their skulls, and were prescribed immunosuppressive drugs. In the sham condition, the dura, a thick membrane surrounding the brain, was not penetrated. Disturbingly, a year after the surgeries, no statistically significant difference in clinical benefit was found between the verum and sham surgery groups.

Ethical Issues and Other Challenges

Sham surgery is, by its very nature, an invasive placebo control involving the use of anesthesia and incisions. In the fetal transplantation studies, ethicists argued that the risks to those who received the sham intervention outweighed any potential scientific or societal benefit. Possible complications from anesthesia include nerve injury, allergic reactions, nausea, vomiting, and malignant hyperthermia. Incisions put the patient at risk for increased pain, bleeding, and/or infection. Given the risks to patients, some ethicists have contended that sham surgery is intrinsically or presumptively unethical, and violates the ethical imperative to "do no harm."

In addition to the ethical challenges, executing a sham surgery can be costly and engage many clinical confederates to provide a convincing scene in the surgical theater. In sham surgeries, confederates must replicate audiovisual (e.g., dialogue between surgeons and technicians) and olfactory (e.g., the distinct smell of the polymer used in vertebroplasty) cues. In addition, props such as suction devices, catheters, infusion pumps, and even dark goggles to literally blind the patients can be required.

Logistically, surgery is expensive, and it is unusual for funding bodies to be motivated to fund a placebo-controlled clinical trial unless it is to test the safety of a new marketable device. Given the propensity for clinical trials with low enrollment to drag on past their funding period, and be abandoned or unpublished, the possibility of risk exposure to subjects and financial loss with no guaranteed benefit to society is a constant concern.[9]

Recent Studies That Compared Surgery to Sham Surgery

A landmark study in 2002 reinvigorated the ethical debate and ushered in the modern era of placebo-controlled surgery trials. J. Bruce Moseley and colleagues randomized 180 patients with knee osteoarthritis to either arthroscopic debridement (a minor surgery to remove damaged bits of bone and cartilage), arthroscopic lavage (a minor surgery using saline to wash out the excess fluid or debris in the joint), or sham surgery. The outcomes were assessed over a twenty-four-month period. Cited by subsequent academic articles over twenty-five hundred times, the *New England Journal of Medicine* report of this trial would capture the attention of modern surgeons and health care quality experts. Once again, in a sham-controlled trial of an expensive and widely popular surgery, the researchers found that "at no point did either of the intervention groups report less pain or better function than the placebo group."[10] More recently, a meta-analysis comparing arthroscopic surgery to nonsurgical interventions like exercise, physical therapy, or steroid injection suggested that arthroscopic surgery is not more effective than the less invasive alternatives.[11]

Another widely publicized series of sham-controlled surgical trials centered around renal denervation for the treatment of resistant hypertension. Resistant hypertension is characterized by a failure to respond to three or more antihypertensive drugs. Surprisingly, there are nontrivial placebo effects in patients with resistant and nonresistant hypertension.[12] In renal denervation, nerves in the wall of the renal artery are ablated by radiofrequency pulses or an ultrasound, causing a reduction in sympathetic neuronal activity and decrease in blood pressure. The early trials of the Symplicity Catheter System, Symplicity HTN-1, 2009, and HTN-2, 2010, were single-armed trials with promising results. In Symplicity HTN-3, however, a sham-controlled trial performed in 2017, no difference was observed between the blood pressure reduction from verum denervation, −14 mmHg, and the sham control, −11mmHg, six months after the surgeries. Undaunted by these disappointing results, the manufacturers of the Symplicity denervation device continued to perfect the target, number of ablation points, and selection of participants to see if these factors influenced the benefit of the treatment over a placebo. Notwithstanding these technical improvements, the benefit of renal denervation is still only modestly better than a placebo.[13]

Yet if either surgery or its sham equivalent ameliorate a patient's symptoms, when neither wins, should we take both off the table?

Cutting to the Chase

There is a large body of evidence supporting what was long suspected by Beecher and others: that some surgeries, steeped as they are in ritual, are potent inducers of placebo effects. A 2014 review of placebo-controlled surgery trials found improvement in patients randomized to a placebo in 74 percent of the trials, and no difference between surgery and a placebo in 15 percent of the trials.[14] In 49 percent of the trials, the surgery had a greater effect than a placebo, but the magnitude of this difference was small.

If the last sixty-plus years are viewed with a societal lens, one might argue that discrediting popular surgeries like mammary artery ligation and more recently renal denervation as shams and removing them from the surgeon's arsenal saved thousands of people from undergoing a useless surgery.[15] But the question of whether a surgery works or not isn't a simple open-and-shut case. Yes, many popular surgeries, when tested in sham-controlled trials, proved to be no better than a placebo. Yet if either surgery or its sham equivalent ameliorate a patient's symptoms, when neither wins, should we take both off the table? Shouldn't we offer at least one of these approaches to the patient? With 150,000 patients in the United Kingdom and 700,000 in the United States still undergoing knee arthroscopies annually, perhaps at least some of these surgeries, effective or not, are still on the table.[16]

WHO RESPONDS?

We found that there were no differences in sex ratios or in intelligence between reactors and nonreactors. There are however significant differences in attitudes, habits, educational background, and personality structure between consistent reactors and nonreactors.

—Henry Beecher, "The Powerful Placebo," 1955

The Placebo Reactor

The question of who responds to a placebo treatment is a complex one. While the answer could revolutionize clinical care and drug development, this question is not top of mind among clinicians, drug developers ignore it until it's too late, and academic placebo researchers tend to tackle the problem from their respective vantage points. Placebo psychologists look for answers in behavioral and personality differences, placebo neuroscientists look for brain signatures, and placebo geneticists seek genetic variants. More recently, interdisciplinary studies aided by machine learning (a type of artificial intelligence that learns from data and can identify patterns) are combining psychological, neurobiological, and genetic perspectives to predict who will respond to placebos in clinical trials.

As clinical trials increasingly fail to beat placebos, the race to identify predictive features becomes more urgent. Such prediction tools are becoming more attractive to trialists, and drug developers are seeking to beat placebos and counteract the threat to drug development that they pose. Several of these methods are patented and form the basis for companies. But how well do these prediction methods work, and how can physicians and drug developers use them effectively? In this chapter, I focus on what we know about placebo responders, and consider the options and subsequent challenges for what we will do when we can accurately predict who responds.

Is There a Placebo Responder Personality Type?

The short answer is not really. Findings across the scores of studies looking at personality and placebo responders have not been consistent. This is in large part due to the small study sizes with large heterogeneity across participants as well as the experimental and clinical conditions. Study participants vary by age, sex, geographic location, health status (i.e., healthy or a patient), and disease severity. Study protocols can vary by the duration of treatment, dosage, delivery of the intervention (i.e., pill or surgery), study details conveyed in the informed consent, phase of the trial, attitude and bedside manner of the clinician, and so on. Added to this is the tension in academics between the pressure to produce innovative, exploratory work, and the necessity to replicate and validate previous findings before they can be translated to clinical practices. Thus grants and journals put a premium on novelty. Replicating a finding once or twice to validate a result is important. Beyond that, repeating the same study over and over again is considered a crisis of creativity. So we have a lot of small studies that examine numerous experimental models across healthy controls and clinical conditions, making the translation of these findings to clinical practices tedious and currently beyond reach.

Psychological Markers of the Placebo Responder

You might argue that if there was a common placebo personality type, it would emerge despite the heterogeneity, but this hasn't happened. Still, in the field of personality of placebo responders, there are some important and intriguing trends. The "big five" is a way of categorizing broad personality traits. The five traits are: *openness to experience*, which describes people who tend to be inventive and curious as opposed to consistent and cautious; *extraversion*, which captures people who are outgoing and energetic versus solitary and reserved; *agreeableness*, which portrays people who are friendly and compassionate versus critical and rational; *conscientiousness*, which is associated with people who are efficient and organized versus extravagant and careless; and *neuroticism*, which relates to people who are sensitive and nervous versus resilient and confident. Of the big five personality factors, openness to experience and extraversion are the two most frequently observed in placebo studies.[1]

Optimism and pessimism represent the two ends of another useful personality scale: the life orientation test. Dispositional optimism, which measures a generalized positive outcome expectancy for the future, is often associated with a placebo response.[2] Conversely, pessimism, which measures a tendency to have negative expectations about the future, is associated with a nocebo response.[3] Several other psychological traits have been examined in placebo studies, but few have been replicated. Among these studies, suggestibility, expectation, and a desire for relief were also found to be more prevalent in participants who respond to a placebo.

A dynamic transactional model was proposed as one way to better use personality traits to predict and understand placebo responses. In this model, personality traits are grouped into two constructs: "inward" and "outward." Inward traits, like suggestibility, absorption, and acquiescence, are associated with greater sensitivity to interior states (how one feels inside). Outward traits, like extraversion, optimism, altruism, and ego resiliency, are associated with a greater permeability to external input. In this dynamic transactional model, individuals would be more or less sensitive to a given placebo treatment depending on the context and environmental cues associated with the treatment. The applicability of the dynamic transactional model is exemplified in a clinical trial in IBS that looked at three "doses" of a placebo and found that the outward trait of extraversion was associated with only one type of placebo treatment.[4]

What Does Neuroimaging Tell Us about Placebo Responders?

The observation that the positive effect of a practitioner can have a greater effect on a patient's symptoms as compared to a placebo alone is not new, but it suggests that at least in part, a placebo response is a state—a temporary way of being (e.g., hungry), rather than a trait, or a more stable and enduring feature (e.g., eye color). Still, there is good evidence that brain structure and connectivity—traits that are amenable to change over time—can predict a placebo response.

Modern neuroimaging techniques allow for the identification of some of these structural and functional differences that can underlie the responsiveness to treatment. One such technique, functional connectivity, is based on fMRI, and utilizes the magnetic properties of hemoglobin to image changes in blood flow that co-occur with activity to evaluate the extent to which regions are functionally connected. In these studies, the implication is that regions that are active simultaneously, or are "coactivated," are connected to each other, serving as a proxy for "connectivity." In a series of two studies of patients with chronic knee osteoarthritis, neural connectivity during pain exposure was found to predict a placebo response.[5] The greatest difference between responders and nonresponders was the magnitude of connectivity between the right middle frontal gyrus, a prefrontal cortical region involved in decision-making, memory, and planning, and the rest of the brain.

Using Computational Tools to Predict Placebo Responders

With the recognition that a placebo response is multifactorial, the quest for tools to predict placebo responders turned to using composite scores and machine learning to identify combinations of demographic, psychological, and neuroimaging measures that prospectively predict who responds to a placebo.

One study of patients with chronic lower back pain used machine learning to find combinations of neural or psychological traits that predicted responses to taking placebo pills.[6] The participants were randomized to blinded placebo pills or no treatment, and asked to report their back pain on a phone app over the fifteen months of the study. The placebo pill patients had greater improvements in pain intensity compared to the no-pill control participants. None of the traditional psychological measures typically observed in experimental pain studies predicted the treatment response. Instead, the placebo response was predicted by the combined effect of subscales related to openness, emotional awareness, the ability to describe inner experience, sensitivity to nonpainful situations, and reduced distraction about pain and discomfort.

In the same study, neuroimaging data obtained at the baseline, before the participants were randomly sorted into groups, showed that there were differences in anatomy and connectivity in the brain that could predict placebo responses. Some of these features included cortical thickness in sensorimotor-related regions, volume asymmetry in subcortical areas, and connectivity differences between pain-associated areas, including parts of the

PFC, ACC, and PAG. While the psychological and neurological models were independently predictive of placebo responses, they were not correlated, and the addition of imaging to the psychological data did not improve the predictability of the model. Thus, while it would be simpler and certainly less expensive to use a psychological test as a proxy for the neuroanatomical and neurophysiological biomarkers, this last observation suggests that these measures are predictive of distinct elements but not placebo responses as a whole.

In another study using machine learning to model placebo reactors, education was found to be a strong predictor of placebo responses in patients with late-life depression.[7] In this study, among those patients with more than twelve years of education, the placebo almost outperformed the active medication. In another study of depression in adolescent patients, the placebo response was predicted by a composite score of sex, age, being nonwhite, having a history of depression, and the baseline depression score.[8] Machine learning requires large data sets, and because of the preponderance of small studies, replication of these findings in the short term is unlikely. In many studies, the baseline disease severity score is a strong predictor of a response to placebo treatment.[9] This is quite likely because patients seek help and are willing to enroll in clinical trials when their symptoms are at their worst. While this might seem like it is just regression to the mean, in many cases controlling for the baseline symptom severity does not eliminate the whole effect of a placebo treatment.

Genetics and the Placebo Response: The Garbage Gene

Enzymes are a type of protein that carry out chemical reactions in the body. Catechol-O-methyltransferase (COMT) is the major enzyme that eliminates dopamine in the PFC, one of the regions activated with a placebo treatment. As discussed in the chapter on the neurobiology of placebo responses (chapter 3), dopamine signaling is induced in some participants who respond to a placebo treatment. Most of this signaling takes place in the PFC. One hypothesis is that if variation in the COMT gene influences the dopamine function in the PFC, it could influence a response to a placebo treatment too. The COMT protein also metabolizes neurotransmitters and hormones that are important in the cardiovascular, autonomic nervous, and endocrine systems. COMT effects are so frequently observed in psychological, neurological, cardiovascular, and even a few cancer studies that some researchers dubbed it the "garbage gene." But a garbage gene that, like placebos, is associated with many outcomes across many conditions, is precisely what one might look for in a placebo gene.

Genes are made up of four different molecules called nucleotides, abbreviated as A, C, T, and G. The combinations of these nucleotides across our twenty-three pairs of chromosomes make up the genetic code. Small changes in the nucleotide sequence called polymorphisms can change the way a gene, or the protein it makes, functions. These changes happen in nature all the time. A majority of them are not harmful and simply add to human diversity. Sometimes these small changes can have more subtle effects. Though the findings are inconsistent, there is some evidence that genetics might influence some behavior, like the responsiveness to a placebo.

A common single nucleotide polymorphism in the COMT gene called rs4680 changes a G nucleotide to an A around the middle of the gene. This change results in two different versions of the gene and the proteins they encode. The valine (val) version is more efficient at metabolizing dopamine than the methionine (met) version. Hence individuals who are homozygous for the val version of the enzyme (val/val) break down dopamine three to four times more efficiently than individuals who are homozygous for the met (met/met) version. As a result, met/met individuals tend to have more dopamine available in their PFC than val/val ones.[10] Heterozygous individuals, val/met, have an intermediate level of PFC dopamine.

In an IBS study examining the relationship between a placebo response and the COMT genotype among three placebo treatment arms (no treatment, sham acupuncture alone, or sham acupuncture plus a supportive clinician-patient interaction), met/met participants were found to have a greater placebo response than val/met and val/val participants, and this difference was greatest in the supportive treatment arm.[11] This finding was replicated in a recent IBS clinical trial in which met/met participants had a greater response to double-blind placebo pills than val/met and val/val participants (figure 10).[12]

Gene-Drug Interactions

> We can take an example from our own work
> where placebos have relieved pain arising from
> physiological cause (surgical incision) and show
> how useful the screening out of reactors can be.
> I, with Keats, Mosteller, and Lasagna, in 1953,
> administered analgesics by mouth to patients having
> steady, severe, postoperative wound pain, and we
> found that when we took all patients and all data we
> could not differentiate between certain combined
> acetylsalicylic acid data and narcotic (morphine and
> codeine) data; however, when we screened out the
> placebo reactors, a sharp differential emerged in
> favor of the acetylsalicylic acid administered orally as
> opposed to the narcotics administered orally.
>
> —Henry Beecher, "The Powerful Placebo," 1955

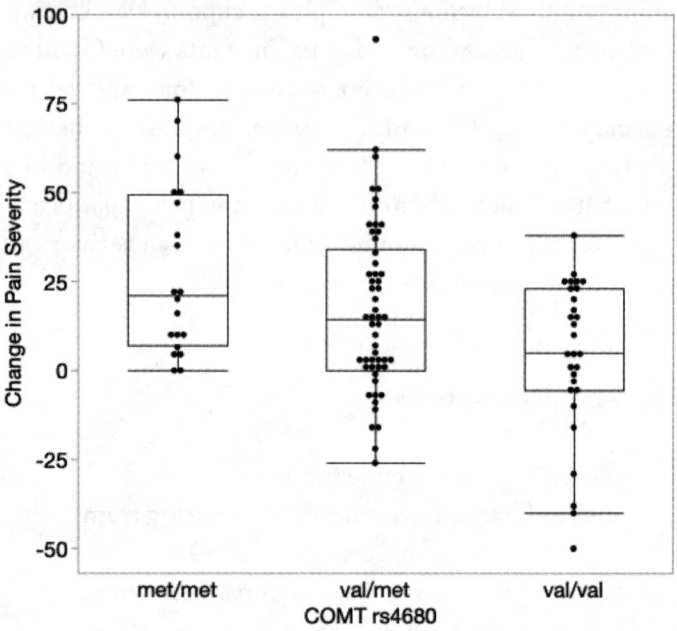

Figure 10 The genetic variation in COMT rs4680 (val158met) is associated with a differential response to a placebo treatment in IBS. *Source:* J. Vollert, R. Wang, S. Regis, H. E. Yetman, A. Lembo, T. Kaptchuk, V. Cheng, et al., "Genotypes of Pain and Analgesia in a Randomized Trial of Irritable Bowel Syndrome," *Frontiers in Psychiatry* 23 (March 2022), https://www.frontiersin .org/articles/10.3389/fpsyt.2022.842030/full.

COMT rs4680 effects are not limited to placebo treatment in IBS. The association with a response to a placebo treatment has been observed across several conditions. Interestingly, the directions of these effects not only differ across conditions but also appear to be further modified by some drugs. Examples of this include trials of tolcapone for memory, propranolol for pain, clonidine for chronic fatigue syndrome (figure 11), aspirin for cardiovascular disease prevention, and vitamin E for cancer prevention.[13] In these studies, the direction of the effect differs by the treatment arm such that in some studies, the met/met participants respond to a placebo but do worse on a drug. In other studies, the val/val participants do better on a placebo but worse on a drug. Because clinical trials typically compare the average effects in the active and placebo treatment arms, these differential results are masked when we only consider the net effects in the drug and placebo arms.

One of the fundamental assumptions of the randomized placebo-controlled clinical trial is that the drug and placebo responses are additive. That is why we can simply subtract the clinical outcome in the placebo arm from that observed in the drug treatment arm to determine the efficacy of the treatment. But what if in addition to naloxone, there are other drugs that perturb the placebo response? And what if, as we saw here with the COMT gene and

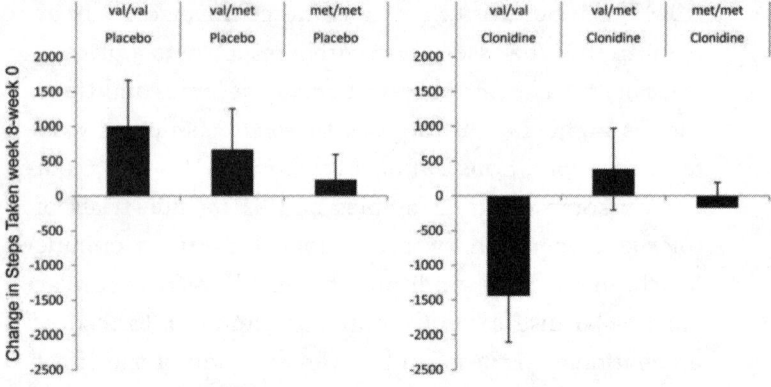

Figure 11 In patients with chronic fatigue syndrome, the change between the baseline and outcome after an eight-week treatment is plotted by COMT genotype and treatment type. *Source*: K. T. Hall, J. Kossowsky, T. F. Oberlander, T. J. Kaptchuk, J. P. Saul, V. B. Wyller, E. Fagermoen, et al., "Genetic Variation in Catechol-O-methyltransferase Modifies Effects of Clonidine Treatment in Chronic Fatigue Syndrome," *Pharmacogenomics Journal* 16, no. 5 (October 2016): 454–460, https://doi.org/10.1038/tpj.2016.53.

tolcapone, propranolol, clonidine, aspirin, and vitamin E, this pharmacogenomic effect varies depending on the genotype, disease or condition, and drug being studied? Could differential pharmacogenomic effects in the drug and placebo arms mask the true effect of the drugs in genetically defined subpopulations? These pharmacogenomic interactions and their influence on outcomes in clinical trials are precisely what precision medicine is designed to address. To date, however, precision medicine has failed to fully account for the contribution of genetic effects in the placebo arms of clinical trials. Perhaps it's time for us to critically examine the potential for these placebo-related gene-drug interactions to influence how we determine the efficacy of drugs.

A placebo response, as we are learning, is a complex phenotype, and in addition to the many demographic and psychological variables that might influence a placebo response, there are likely many other genes that contribute to this outcome. Although placebo genomics is in its infancy, a review of the literature shows that there are already many other genes that influence outcomes in the placebo arms of clinical trials and potentially interact with the drug being tested. In network medicine, proteins with similar functions form modules with distinct properties that can shed light on their mutual function. Network analyses of the proteins encoded by genes that influence a placebo response, termed the *placebome* (genes or the proteins that they encode that influence a placebo response), can be identified in the network of all known proteins called the interactome. The placebome module, or genetic subnetwork, appears to be proximal and sometimes overlaps with diseases and conditions known to have high placebo response rates. The placebome also maps proximal to modules of several drug classes, providing one explanation for why so many drugs appear to perturb the placebo response (figure 12).[14]

Perhaps it's time for us to critically examine the potential for these placebo-related gene-drug interactions to influence how we determine the efficacy of drugs.

		Placebome module	
Drug categories	**Size of the targets**	**Proximity**	**P**
Analgesics, non-narcotic	142	0.96	3.5×10^{-10}
Appetite depressants	88	1.04	1.78×10^{-12}
Antidepressive agents	262	1.04	8.6×10^{-5}
Sympathomimetics	165	1.07	2.6×10^{-6}
Antiparkinson agents	179	1.07	6.0×10^{-6}
Cardiotonic agents	72	1.09	1.2×10^{-11}
Serotonin uptake inhibitors	140	1.11	6.5×10^{-7}
Central nervous system depressants	78	1.13	6.1×10^{-9}
Antioxidants	116	1.19	1.4×10^{-5}
Dopamine agents	78	1.22	6.5×10^{-7}
Excitatory amino acid antagonists	99	1.22	1.5×10^{-5}
Dopamine uptake inhibitors	74	1.30	1.7×10^{-5}
Adrenergic α-agonists	126	1.30	9.1×10^{-3}
Neuroprotective agents	43	1.31	2.5×10^{-7}
Adrenergic β-agonists	28	1.50	3.1×10^{-4}

Figure 12 This table shows drug target categories that are significantly proximate to the placebome module in the human interactome. *Note: P* values were adjusted using the Bonferroni procedure. *Source:* R. S. Wang, K. T. Hall, F. Giulianini, D. Passow, T. J. Kaptchuk, and J. Loscalzo, "Network Analysis of the Genomic Basis of the Placebo Effect," *JCI Insight* 2, no. 11 (June 2, 2017), https://doi.org/10.1172/jci.insight.93911.

If We Could Predict Placebo Responders, What Would We Do Next?

While identifying predictors of the placebo response is vital to understanding who may benefit from a placebo treatment and improving the design of clinical trials, the use of such a tool invites several questions and potential ethical concerns. If we identified a subset of the population that responded to placebos, would it be excluded from clinical trials? If this subset was excluded, would the drugs that get developed based on these trials require a black box label? And if this was the case, what drugs would we prescribe to placebo responders? Would it be ethical for them to receive a placebo? Would they have to be told that they are placebo responders? If we told them they were placebo responders, would that change the nature of their response? If one is a placebo responder in a depression trial, would they be one for a hypertension trial? Once a placebo responder, are you always a placebo responder? What group of genes influence a placebo response, and are there gene-gene as well as gene-drug interactions? Which drugs perturb a placebo response? Can we use drugs to boost a placebo response?

Clearly there are many questions we can ask. With evidence in some conditions that the placebo response is increasing in clinical trials, it likely means that there is more to the placebo response than the stable traits of genetics and brain structure. But who will invest time and resources into addressing these questions?

PLACEBO REDUX

The success of medical practice essentially depends
upon the faculty of sagacious discernment. One
who is carried away by every wind of doctrine, and
who recommends every new medicine which is in
vogue and becomes popular, without considering
the evidence and fair probability of its efficacy,
will frequently administer mort, and sometimes
injurious remedies, to his patients.

—John Haygarth, *Of the Imagination*, January 1, 1800

Over two hundred years have passed since Franklin de-
bunked Mesmer, and Haygarth did the same to Perkins,
publishing *Of the Imagination, as a Cause and as a Cure of
Disorders of the Body*. During that time, the developments
in psychological, pharmacological, neurobiological, and genetic studies of placebo effects have done much to broaden
our understanding of their full complexity. Still, we resist

acknowledging their power. Perhaps this is because of the centrality of mechanism in explaining the action of drugs. We identify pathways perturbed in disease, design drugs that target these pathways, and conduct animal studies and clinical trials to derive evidence in patients that these interventions work. Yet many diligently designed and developed compounds fail to demonstrate efficacy beyond that of a placebo.

In creating justifications for these failures, we invariably attribute them to the wrong dose, wrong patient demographic, or wrong outcome measure. In so doing, we seek to layer objectivity over results we don't quite understand and cannot quite control. By invoking a mechanism of failure, we are back on even footing and can try again.

In focusing on why the drug failed, we are missing that other mechanism, the one that didn't fail. This other mechanism gives rise to placebo effects. Via brain regions like the vmPFC, this mechanism attaches meaning, expectations, and in turn a neurological response to stimuli. Armed with a mechanism, placebos are finally moving, albeit slowly, into that privileged space of cause and biological effect.

Placebos in the Time of COVID-19

The COVID-19 pandemic inadvertently highlighted the real-life powers and limitations of placebo as well as nocebo effects. Notably, placebos were no match for the virus. For example, no matter how much we wished, prayed, or expected that hydroxychloroquine would work, it didn't.[1] After several placebo-controlled clinical trials, it was clear that hydroxychloroquine, like placebos, was no match for the virus. Despite the urgent need to counteract SARS-CoV-2, the virus that causes COVID-19, promising vaccines and antiviral drugs like remdesivir all had to first demonstrate safety and efficacy beyond a placebo before being made publicly available.[2]

SARS-CoV-2 has taken over six million lives worldwide as of this writing. At the same time, nocebos and powerful negative expectations are everywhere. Notwithstanding evidence that face masks could greatly reduce the spread of the virus, wearing them became a political statement instead of a prophylactic measure. While vaccines with demonstrated effectiveness are almost universally available, vaccine hesitancy as a result of negative information has greatly reduced people's willingness to be vaccinated. On an individual level, as we saw throughout this book, negative information can shape personal beliefs and expectations, which in turn result in adverse effects and poor treatment adherence. What COVID-19 showed us was that on a population level, negative information and its downstream nocebo effects can compromise our public health with devastating health, social, and economic repercussions.

Mitigating Clinical Trial Failure

If and when the COVID-19 pandemic finally ends, and we emerge from behind our masks and sheltering places, we will have to deal with the many challenges that faced us before. Pain and depression will still be with us, and so too the challenges of developing novel effective neuro-psych drugs. Quite likely, novel treatments that are only as efficacious as a placebo will continue to fail. To counteract this trend, numerous strategies are on the horizon, from educating participants and investigators about the placebo response, to the development of machine learning algorithms to predict placebo responders and digital therapeutics that promise to revolutionize medicine. Even the possibility of using placebos to treat patients is back on the table.

If You Can't Beat Them, Prescribe Them: Open-Label Placebos

With demonstrated clinical benefits in numerous conditions over the seventy-five years of clinical trials, and now a confirmed and compelling mechanism of action, one might wonder why we have not deployed placebos as treatments in modern clinical medicine. Although deemed unethical according to central tenets of patient autonomy, several studies suggest that use of placebos by physicians is still widespread.[3] Some physicians report using impure placebos (low doses of an active treatment, vitamin, or supplement), and in countries like Canada, Portugal, and Germany, pure placebos like sugar pills or saline injections are prevalent.[4] In fact, Germany has gone one step further. In 2012, the German Medical Association, after careful assessment and deliberation, concluded that the use of placebos in clinical practice was justified.[5] Specifically, the scientific advisory board found that placebo use was "acceptable" in three circumstances: for patients with a minor condition, when there is no other effective treatment available, and when treatment with a placebo is likely to succeed. Not surprisingly, this announcement was met with trepidation from concerned bioethicists who worried that patients' rights were being violated. As this debate continues, researchers have taken the unprecedented step of breaking the blind. Now, in over a dozen trials, patients have been treated with an open-label placebo (OLP), or a placebo without deception.

OLP clinical trials have demonstrated that clinical benefit from a placebo treatment can be preserved with OLPs or honestly prescribed placebos.[6] In randomized clinical trials of conditions such as chronic low back pain, cancer-related fatigue, IBS, and allergic rhinitis, patients reported significant benefit from OLPs compared to no treatment or care-as-usual controls.[7] The theory of how OLPs work builds on the placebo neuroimaging studies and predictive coding theories discussed earlier in this book. Briefly, the brain uses prediction processing to reassess incoming information in favor of the clinical improvement of symptoms.[8] The honest information conveyed by the physician about the potential of the placebo treatment to improve the condition of the patient supports this reassessment, seeding a shift in the perception of symptoms.

OLPs work best when administered with the clinician sharing the plausible rationale of how placebos work and an overview of the positive effects of placebos in previous clinical trials. Additionally, physicians are encouraged to allow the patient to suspend belief while creating an openness to the possibility, but not an absolute certainty, that the placebo pills might work. The key instruction to patients is that they must adhere to the treatment. The ritual of pill taking thus promotes a top-down revision of the patient's perception of their condition as moving toward symptom relief. More OLP trials are ongoing, and although these trials are small, their demonstration of efficacy to date is striking and suggests a path forward to once again using placebos in the clinic to benefit patients.

Placebos are not just being leveraged in the clinic. ZEEBO and the XPILL are trademarked placebos that are commercially available direct to consumers over the internet. Although they have not been tested in clinical trials, it is likely that they will do as well as a number of placebos.

Placebos . . . There's an App for That

Smartphones, the "Pac-Men" of the electronics industry, gobbled up cameras, radios, clocks, and calculators. Now that gaping mouth is set on the pharmaceutical industry. As of June 2020, AKL-T01, having gone through clinical trials and regulatory review, is now an FDA-approved prescription treatment for attention deficit and hyperactivity in children. But AKL-T01 is not a pill; it's a video game. Trademarked EndeavorRx, AKL-T01 joins the growing number of digiceuticals, or digital health technologies, that coach patients to manage their conditions while tracking medication intake, lifestyle, behavior, food intake, and physical activity. The clinical trial results for these interventions are generally quite impressive. In the case of AKL-T01, patients randomized to the active intervention had significant improvement in the test of variables of attention with minimal adverse events compared to a control app, which in this case was a word puzzle.[9]

Digital health technologies now have their own specialty academic journals, like *Lancet Digital Health*, to manage and publish the outflow of research in this relatively new field. Virtual reality has also emerged as a platform with promising results in the treatment of psychiatric illnesses as well as chronic and acute pain.[10] Still, many initial trials of virtual reality interventions are thought to be lacking in rigorous scientific methodology, and do not tend to include a placebo control, or for that matter, any control.[11]

As these fields develop, factors that influence clinical outcomes like sample size, clinically relevant measures, and what represents an acceptable comparator or placebo control have to be addressed.[12] When it comes to interventions administered through virtual reality or other digital mechanisms, the line between a device and placebo control can be blurred, and we will need to identify the "active" elements. Is it the device, a given image, or the application that brings this all together?

Slamming the Back Door

From benign patriarchal palliative to quackery and clinical trial control, placebos have played many roles in the history of medicine. In many guises as bread pills, metal rods, sugar pills, or sham surgery, theirs has been a command performance. However inert the placebo, their administration has striking ameliorative properties—the placebo's paradox. This ability of placebos to reduce suffering from a myriad of symptoms is intricately linked to the symbols and rituals that over centuries were enlisted in the service of healing. In contrast, negative verbal or contextual information induce negative expectations, and whether intentional or unintentional, are coded to elicit harm.

With the identification of neurological drivers of placebo effects, the curtain has been pulled back, and the stigma and mystery are giving way to mechanism. As I discussed throughout this book, placebo treatment can access neural processes linked to brain regions like the vmPFC that can in a top-down fashion reshape our experience of incoming signals based on positive (placebo) or negative (nocebo) expectations. Thus placebo effects along with their opposite, nocebo effects, represent a back door to the amelioration or exacerbation of the experience of pain and other negative symptoms.

Given this potential for benefit or harm, the clinician, as trusted healer, the person we go to in our hour (or all too frequently, only fifteen minutes) of need, has an ethical responsibility to safeguard this back door. As I examined in this book, this has not always been the case. When medicine was more patriarchal, an "all-knowing" physician could prescribe an "impure placebo," a treatment for patients who had exhausted all possible known treatments. But the back door is known to many, and we were and are all too vulnerable to the promises of quacks as well as today's carefully crafted social media messages designed to control our beliefs and attitudes about our health.

Clinicians, researchers, drug developers, and patients all have differing opinions on placebos. By now you have probably formed your own opinion on the benefit, harm, uselessness, or utility of placebos and the placebo effect.

Safeguarding the
back door is the work
of us all.

Of one thing we can be certain: no matter how we see them, placebos represent what was for many years ignored, hidden, or wild, but was always a back door to influencing our health and wellness. Through the pages of this book, we have seen the mechanism underlying placebo effects used in the service of healing and the propagation of harms. How we use this at once new and ancient mechanism is not only up to clinicians and clinical trialists. Safeguarding the back door is the work of us all.

ACKNOWLEDGMENTS

To Keats and Hyacinth, whose words are my constant guides.

This book would not have been possible without my intrepid research assistant, Hailey Yetman, who tolerated my erratic schedule and complete disregard for commas. I am indebted to Vicki Garcia, Helen Klonaris, Dominique Hall, Ted Kaptchuk, Joseph Loscalzo, Elisabeth Battinelli, Anthony Lembo, Mabel Smith, Peter Wayne, JoAnn Manson, Ruisheng Wang, Jocelyn Silvester, Elberta Stone, Allyson Sherlock, Gloria Yeh, Mary Anne Ryan, Matthew Browne, Daniel Chasman, Irving Kirsch, and Kenneth Mukamal, whose insights were critical to telling this story of placebos. Thank you Hesam Dashti for sharing the story of your grandmother and her lifesaving placebo treatments.

Special thanks to Valerie Stone whose love and support kept me grounded throughout this journey, and to my dog, Placebo, who was a constant companion through many late nights.

Agonist
A molecule that interacts with and activates a receptor.

Amphetamine
A synthetic drug that has a stimulant effect. Used to treat attention deficit and hyperactivity as well as and narcolepsy.

Analgesia
Relief of pain or state of being insensitive to pain.

Antagonist
A molecule that interacts with and deactivates or inhibits a receptor.

Blinding
Concealing group assignment or some other feature of treatment (i.e., whether patients are randomized to a placebo or active treatment) that might influence the outcomes from the participants.

Carfentanil
A strong synthetic opioid. In PET studies, radioactively tagged carfentanil ($[^{11}C]$-carfentanil) can be used to track mu-opioid receptor activity in the brain.

Conditioning
Training, consciously or unconsciously, a person or animal to associate a certain stimulus with a certain response.

Connectivity
Connectivity in neuroimaging refers to temporal correlations between two structures that suggest that these structures directionally or bidirectionally influence each other.

Dopamine
A neurotransmitter that is associated with signaling in reward, motivation, and motor pathways. Dopamine pathway dysfunction is implicated in multiple diseases and illnesses, including substance misuse or addiction, schizophrenia, attention deficit and hyperactivity, Parkinson's disease, and others.

Double-blind
In a clinical trial, concealing the group assignment or some other feature of treatment (i.e., whether patients are randomized to a placebo or active treatment) that might influence the outcomes from both participants and experimenters.

Endogenous opioids
Opioid peptides that naturally occur in the brain and interact with opioid receptors to relieve pain and signal reward.

Functional magnetic resonance imaging (fMRI)
An imaging technique that utilizes the magnetic properties of hemoglobin to generate images of the brain based on blood flow. An fMRI can be used to create contrasts that show differences in brain activity at different times.

Hawthorne effects
Effects that occur simply because a subject is being observed in a study.

Hyperalgesia
Increase of pain or state of being hypersensitive to pain.

Meta-analysis
An analysis of results from multiple studies.

Naloxone
An opioid antagonist that is commonly used to block the effects of opioids during an overdose.

Natural history
The natural course of a disease or illness in an individual, starting from onset, peaking, and then resolving.

Nocebo effects
Negative or adverse events or effects that occur in response to an inert or placebo treatment.

Nociceptive pain
Short-term pain that originates from the activation of nociceptors with damage of tissue.

Nociceptor
A sensory receptor that responds to painful stimuli.

No treatment control
A control group in which the participants receive no treatment at all to serve as a neutral comparison to other treatments.

Open-label placebo (OLP)
Placebos that are administered openly or without deception.

Perkins's tractors
Small metal rods patented by Elisha Perkins as a "cure-all."

Pharmacogenomics
The study of how genome variation is associated with an individual drug treatment response with the aim of improving the development of safer and more efficacious drugs. Pharmacogenomics is a key field of study in the pursuit of personalized or precision medicine.

Placebo effects
Events or effects that occur in response to an inert or placebo treatment.

Placebome
The group of genome-related or genome-derived molecules that are hypothesized to affect an individual's placebo response. Some of these molecules may include genes, proteins, and microRNAs, among others.

Positron emission tomography (PET)
An imaging technique that utilizes the properties of radioactive particles to create images of the human body. A PET scan be used to differentiate between tissue types, and in neuroscience, it can be used to observe cerebral blood flow or receptor activity.

Prediction error
The mismatch between what was expected and what actually happens. The prediction error is encoded by dopamine signaling and is instrumental to learning. The prediction error is instrumental to learning and, in reward processing, is encoded by dopamine.

Randomized placebo-controlled clinical trial
A clinical trial in which the participants are randomly assigned to active or inert treatment arms in order to test the effectiveness of the active intervention. In a double-blind randomized placebo-controlled clinical trial, the participants are not aware of which treatment arm they have been assigned in order to reduce bias in the reporting outcomes.

Remifentanil
A short-acting synthetic opioid used to relieve pain.

Side effect
An effect, whether positive or negative, that is not the primary intended outcome of a treatment.

Single nucleotide polymorphisms (SNPs)
A site in the genome at which a single nucleotide differs in the DNA nucleotide sequence, causing genetic variability.

Social observational learning
Learning, either conscious or subconscious, that occurs when the observation of behavior of a demonstrator modifies the behavior of the observer.

Statin
A drug used to lower cholesterol levels in the body.

NOTES

Introduction
1. H. H. Moffet, "Sham Acupuncture May Be as Efficacious as True Acupuncture: A Systematic Review of Clinical Trials," *Journal of Alternative and Complementary Medicine* 15, no. 3 (March 2009): 213–216, https://doi.org/10.1089/acm.2008.0356..

2. C. E. Kerr, I. Milne, and T. J. Kaptchuk, "William Cullen and a Missing Mind-Body Link in the Early History of Placebos," *Journal of the Royal Society of Medicine* 101, no. 2 (February 2008): 89–92, https://doi.org/10.1258/jrsm.2007.071005.

3. A. Tinnermann, S. Geuter, C. Sprenger, J. Finsterbusch, and C. Buchel, "Interactions between Brain and Spinal Cord Mediate Value Effects in Nocebo Hyperalgesia," *Science* 358, no. 6359 (October 6, 2017): 105–108, https://doi.org/10.1126/science.aan1221; S. Kam-Hansen, M. Jakubowski, J. M. Kelley, I. Kirsch, D. C. Hoaglin, T. J. Kaptchuk, and R. Burstein, "Altered Placebo and Drug Labeling Changes the Outcome of Episodic Migraine Attacks," *Science Translational Medicine* 6, no. 218 (January 8, 2014): 218ra5. https://doi.org/10.1126/scitranslmed.3006175; K. Faasse and L. R. Martin, "The Power of Labeling in Nocebo Effects," *International Review of Neurobiology* 139 (2018): 379–406, https://doi.org/10.1016/bs.irn.2018.07.016.

4. N. Humphrey, "Great Expectations: The Evolutionary Psychology of Faith-Healing and the Placebo Response," in *Psychology at the Turn of the Millennium: Vol. 2: Social, Developmental, and Clinical Perspectives,* ed. C. von Hofsten and L. Bäckman (Hove, UK: Psychology Press, 2002), 225–246; F. G. Miller, L. Colloca, and T. J. Kaptchuk, "The Placebo Effect: Illness and Interpersonal Healing," *Perspectives in Biology and Medicine* 52, no. 4 (2009): 518–539, https://doi.org/10.1353/pbm.0.0115.

Chapter 1
1. J. Haygarth, *Of the Imagination, as a Cause and as a Cure of Disorders of the Body: Exemplified by Fictitious Tractors and Epidemical Convulsions* (Bath, UK: R. Cruttwell, 1800).

2. C. Booth, "The Rod of Aesculapios: John Haygarth (1740–1827) and Perkins' Metallic Tractors," *Journal of Medical Biography* 13, no. 3 (August 2005): 155–161, https://doi.org/10.1177/096777200501300310.

3. C. E. Kerr, I. Milne, and T. J. Kaptchuk, "William Cullen and a Missing Mind-Body Link in the Early History of Placebos," *Journal of the Royal Society of Medicine* 101, no. 2 (February 2008): 89–92, https://doi.org/10.1258/jrsm.2007.071005.

4. Haygarth, *Of the Imagination*, 2.

5. I. Donaldson, "Royal Commission on Animal Magnetism," 2014, https://www.rcpe.ac.uk/sites/default/files/files/the_royal_commission_on_animal_-_translated_by_iml_donaldson_1.pdf.

6. B. Franklin, *The Autobiography of Benjamin Franklin* (New York: Simon and Schuster, 2004).

7. Haygarth, *Of the Imagination*.

8. J. H. Stewart, "Hypnosis in Contemporary Medicine," *Mayo Clinic Proceedings* 80, no. 4 (April 2005): 511–524, https://doi.org/10.4065/80.4.511.

9. Stewart, "Hypnosis in Contemporary Medicine."

10. I. Loudon, "A Brief History of Homeopathy," *Journal of the Royal Society of Medicine* 99, no. 12 (2006): 607–610. doi:10.1258/jrsm.99.12.607.

11. J. Sliwinski and G. R. Elkins, "Enhancing Placebo Effects: Insights from Social Psychology," *American Journal of Clinical Hypnosis* 55, no. 3 (January 2013): 236–248, https://doi.org/10.1080/00029157.2012.740434; M. Z. Teixeira, C. H. Guedes, P. V. Barreto, and M. A. Martins, "The Placebo Effect and Homeopathy," *Homeopathy* 99, no. 2 (April 2010): 119–129, https://doi.org/10.1016/j.homp.2010.02.001.

12. S. Junod, "FDA and Clinical Drug Trials: A Short History," US Food and Drug Administration, https://www.fda.gov/media/110437/download.

13. Records of the Lydia E. Pinkham Medicine Company, 1776–ca.1985 (inclusive), 1859–1968 (bulk), Schlesinger Library, Radcliffe Institute, Harvard Archives.

14. Richard Cabot, "Truth and Falsehood in Medicine," *Journal of the American Medical Association* 40, no. 15 (1903): 994–994, https://doi.org/10.1001/jama.1903.02490150046006.

15. H. G. Wolff, E. F. Dubois, and H. Gold, "The Use of Placebos in Therapy," *New York State Journal of Medicine* 46 (August 1, 1946): 1718–1727, https://www.ncbi.nlm.nih.gov/pubmed/20993884.

16. C. Carvalho, J. M. Caetano, L. Cunha, P. Rebouta, T. J. Kaptchuk, and I. Kirsch, "Open-Label Placebo Treatment in Chronic Low Back Pain: A Randomized Controlled Trial," *Pain* 157, no. 12 (December 2016): 2766–2772, https://doi.org/10.1097/j.pain.0000000000000700.

17. D. Purves, G. J. Augustine, D. Fitzpatrick, et al., "Central Regulation of Pain Perception," in *Neuroscience*, ed. D. Purves, G. J. Augustine, D. Fitzpatrick,

L. C. Katz, A.-S. LaMantia, J. O. McNamara, and S. M. Williams, chap. 10 (Sunderland, MA: Sinauer Associates, 2001).

18. J. D. Levine, N. C. Gordon, and H. L. Fields, "The Mechanism of Placebo Analgesia," *Lancet* 2, no. 8091 (September 23, 1978): 654–657, https://doi .org/10.1016/s0140-6736(78)92762-9.

19. P. Petrovic, E. Kalso, K. M. Petersson, and M. Ingvar, "Placebo and Opioid Analgesia—Imaging a Shared Neuronal Network," *Science* 295, no. 5560 (March 1, 2002): 1737–1740, https://doi.org/10.1126/science.1067176; T. D. Wager, J. K. Rilling, E. E. Smith, A. Sokolik, K. L. Casey, R. J. Davidson, S. M. Kosslyn, et al., "Placebo-Induced Changes in fMRI in the Anticipation and Experience of Pain," *Science* 303, no. 5661 (February 20, 2004): 1162–1167, https://doi.org/10.1126/science.1093065; H. S. Mayberg, J. A. Silva, S. K. Brannan, J. L. Tekell, R. K. Mahurin, S. McGinnis, and P. A. Jerabek, "The Functional Neuroanatomy of the Placebo Effect," *American Journal of Psychiatry* 159, no. 5 (May 2002): 728–737, https://doi.org/10.1176/ appi.ajp.159.5.728; R. de la Fuente-Fernandez, T. J. Ruth, V. Sossi, M. Schulzer, D. B. Calne, and A. J. Stoessl, "Expectation and Dopamine Release: Mechanism of the Placebo Effect in Parkinson's Disease," *Science* 293, no. 5532 (August 10, 2001): 1164–1166, https://doi.org/10.1126/science. 1060937.

Chapter 2

1. Hesam Dashti, personal communication, November 3, 2021.

2. P. I. Pavlov, "Conditioned Reflexes: An Investigation of the Physiological Activity of the Cerebral Cortex," *Annals of Neuroscience* 17, no. 3 (July 2010): 136–141, https://doi.org/10.5214/ans.0972-7531.1017309.

3. R. J. Herrnstein, "Placebo Effect in the Rat," *Science* 138, no. 3541 (November 9, 1962): 677–678, https://doi.org/10.1126/science.138.3541.677.

4. R. O. Pihl and J. Altman, "An Experimental Analysis of the Placebo Effect," *Journal of Clinical Pharmacology* 11, no. 2 (March–April 1971): 91–95, https:// doi.org/10.1177/009127007101100203.

5. J. M. Danion, S. Peretti, D. Grange, M. Bilik, J. L. Imbs, and L. Singer, "Effects of Chlorpromazine and Lorazepam on Explicit Memory, Repetition Priming and Cognitive Skill Learning in Healthy Volunteers," *Psychopharmacology* 108, no. 3 (1992): 345–351, https://doi.org/10.1007/BF02245122.

6. J. Garcia, W. G. Hankins, J. H. Robinson, and J. L. Vogt, "Bait Shyness: Tests of CS-US Mediation," *Physiology and Behavior* 8, no. 5 (May 1972): 807–810, https://doi.org/10.1016/0031-9384(72)90288-0.

7. R. Ader and N. Cohen, "Behaviorally Conditioned Immunosuppression," *Psychosomatic Medicine* 37, no. 4 (July–August 1975): 333–340, https://www.ncbi.nlm.nih.gov/pubmed/1162023.

8. M. Hadamitzky, L. Luckemann, G. Pacheco-Lopez, and M. Schedlowski, "Pavlovian Conditioning of Immunological and Neuroendocrine Functions," *Physiological Reviews* 100, no. 1 (January 1, 2020): 357–405, https://doi.org/10.1152/physrev.00033.2018.

9. A. Buske-Kirschbaum, C. Kirschbaum, H. Stierle, H. Lehnert, and D. Hellhammer, "Conditioned Increase of Natural Killer Cell Activity (NKCA) in Humans," *Psychosomatic Medicine* 54, no. 2 (March–April 1992): 123–132, https://doi.org/10.1097/00006842-199203000-00001.

10. D. W. Giang, A. D. Goodman, R. B. Schiffer, D. H. Mattson, M. Petrie, N. Cohen, and R. Ader, "Conditioning of Cyclophosphamide-Induced Leukopenia in Humans," *Journal of Neuropsychiatry and Clinical Neurosciences* 8, no. 2 (Spring 1996): 194–201, https://doi.org/10.1176/jnp.8.2.194.

11. L. Colloca, P. Enck, and D. DeGrazia, "Relieving Pain Using Dose-Extending Placebos: A Scoping Review," *Pain* 157, no. 8 (August 2016): 1590–1598, https://doi.org/10.1097/j.pain.0000000000000566.

12. S. Stewart-Williams and J. Podd, "The Placebo Effect: Dissolving the Expectancy versus Conditioning Debate," *Psychological Bulletin* 130, no. 2 (March 2004): 324–340, https://doi.org/10.1037/0033-2909.130.2.324.

13. V. S. Ramachandran and E. L. Altschuler, "The Use of Visual Feedback, in Particular Mirror Visual Feedback, in Restoring Brain Function," *Brain* 132, no. 7 (July 2009): 1693–1710, https://doi.org/10.1093/brain/awp135.

14. J. P. Fisher, D. T. Hassan, and N. O'Connor, "Minerva," *British Medical Journal* 7, no. 310 (1995): 70, https://www.bmj.com/content/310/6971/70.

15. N. Peiris, M. Blasini, T. Wright, and L. Colloca, "The Placebo Phenomenon: A Narrow Focus on Psychological Models," *Perspectives in Biology and Medicine* 61, no. 3 (2018): 388–400, https://doi.org/10.1353/pbm.2018.0051.

16. I. Kirsch, "Response Expectancy and the Placebo Effect," *International Review of Neurobiology* 138 (2018): 81–93, https://doi.org/10.1016/bs.irn.2018.01.003.

17. U. Bingel, V. Wanigasekera, K. Wiech, R. Ni Mhuircheartaigh, M. C. Lee, M. Ploner, and I. Tracey, "The Effect of Treatment Expectation on Drug Efficacy: Imaging the Analgesic Benefit of the Opioid Remifentanil," *Science Translational Medicine* 3, no. 70 (February 16, 2011): 70ra14, https://doi.org/10.1126/scitranslmed.3001244.

18. S. B. Penick and S. Fisher, "Drug-Set Interaction: Psychological and Physiological Effects of Epinephrine under Differential Expectations,"

Psychosomatic Medicine 27 (March–April 1965): 177–182, https://doi
.org/10.1097/00006842-196503000-00010; S. B. Lyerly, S. Ross, A. D. Krug-
man, and D. J. Clyde, "Drugs and Placebos: The Effects of Instructions upon
Performance and Mood under Amphetamine Sulphate and Chloral Hydrate," *Journal of Abnormal Psychology* 68 (March 1964): 321–327, https://
doi.org/10.1037/h0044351; A. J. Dinnerstein and J. Halm, "Modification of
Placebo Effects by Means of Drugs: Effects of Aspirin and Placebos on Self-
Rated Moods," *Journal of Abnormal Psychology* 75, no. 3 (June 1970): 308–314,
https://doi.org/10.1037/h0029313.

19. F. Benedetti, "Placebo and the New Physiology of the Doctor-Patient Relationship," *Physiological Reviews* 93, no. 3 (July 2013): 1207–1246, https://doi
.org/10.1152/physrev.00043.2012.

20. L. Colloca, L. Lopiano, M. Lanotte, and F. Benedetti, "Overt versus Co-
vert Treatment for Pain, Anxiety, and Parkinson's Disease," *Lancet Neurology* 3, no. 11 (November 2004): 679–684, https://doi.org/10.1016/S1474
-4422(04)00908-1.

21. S. Kam-Hansen, M. Jakubowski, J. M. Kelley, I. Kirsch, D. C. Hoaglin, T. J.
Kaptchuk, and R. Burstein, "Altered Placebo and Drug Labeling Changes
the Outcome of Episodic Migraine Attacks," *Science Translational Medicine*
6, no. 218 (January 8, 2014): 218ra5, https://doi.org/10.1126/scitranslmed
.3006175.

22. R. L. Waber, B. Shiv, Z. Carmon, and D. Ariely, "Commercial Features of Placebo and Therapeutic Efficacy," *Journal of the American Medical Association* 299,
no. 9 (March 5, 2008): 1016–1017, https://doi.org/10.1001/jama.299.9.1016;
A. J. Espay, M. M. Norris, J. C. Eliassen, A. Dwivedi, M. S. Smith, C. Banks, J. B.
Allendorfer, et al., "Placebo Effect of Medication Cost in Parkinson Disease: A
Randomized Double-Blind Study," *Neurology* 84, no. 8 (February 24, 2015):
794–802, https://doi.org/10.1212/WNL.0000000000001282.

23. K. Faasse, T. Cundy, G. Gamble, and K. J. Petrie, "The Effect of an Apparent
Change to a Branded or Generic Medication on Drug Effectiveness and Side
Effects," *Psychosomatic Medicine* 75, no. 1 (January 2013): 90–96, https://doi
.org/10.1097/PSY.0b013e3182738826.

24. L. Colloca and F. Benedetti, "Placebo Analgesia Induced by Social Observational Learning," *Pain* 144, no. 1–2 (July 2009): 28–34, https://doi
.org/10.1016/j.pain.2009.01.033.

25. R. A. Wise, S. J. Bartlett, E. D. Brown, M. Castro, R. Cohen, J. T. Holbrook,
C. G. Irvin, et al., "Randomized Trial of the Effect of Drug Presentation on
Asthma Outcomes: The American Lung Association Asthma Clinical Research
Centers," *Journal of Allergy and Clinical Immunology* 124, no. 3 (September
2009): 436–444, https://doi.org/10.1016/j.jaci.2009.05.041.

26. K. R. Sepucha, L. H. Simmons, M. J. Barry, S. Edgman-Levitan, A. M. Licurse, and S. K. Chaguturu, "Ten Years, Forty Decision Aids, and Thousands of Patient Uses: Shared Decision Making at Massachusetts General Hospital," *Health Affairs* 35, no. 4 (April 2016): 630–636, https://doi.org/10.1377/hlthaff.2015.1376.

Chapter 3

1. L. Colloca, D. S. Pine, M. Ernst, F. G. Miller, and C. Grillon, "Vasopressin Boosts Placebo Analgesic Effects in Women: A Randomized Trial," *Biological Psychiatry* 79, no. 10 (May 15, 2016): 794–802, https://doi.org/10.1016/j.biopsych.2015.07.019.

2. R. Melzack, "Evolution of the Neuromatrix Theory of Pain. The Prithvi Raj Lecture: Presented at the Third World Congress of World Institute of Pain, Barcelona 2004," *Pain Practice* 5, no. 2 (June 2005): 85–94, https://doi.org/10.1111/j.1533-2500.2005.05203.x.

3. L. Colloca, *Neurobiology of the Placebo Effect, Part I* (Cambridge, MA: Academic Press, 2018).

4. B. Franklin, *The Autobiography of Benjamin Franklin*. (New York: Simon and Schuster, 2004).

5. P. Petrovic, E. Kalso, K. M. Petersson, and M. Ingvar, "Placebo and Opioid Analgesia—Imaging a Shared Neuronal Network," *Science* 295, no. 5560 (March 1, 2002): 1737–1740, https://doi.org/10.1126/science.1067176; D. J. Scott, C. S. Stohler, C. M. Egnatuk, H. Wang, R. A. Koeppe, and J. K. Zubieta, "Placebo and Nocebo Effects Are Defined by Opposite Opioid and Dopaminergic Responses," *Archives of General Psychiatry* 65, no. 2 (February 2008): 220–231, https://doi.org/10.1001/archgenpsychiatry.2007.34; T. D. Wager, D. J. Scott, and J. K. Zubieta, "Placebo Effects on Human Mu-Opioid Activity during Pain," *Proceedings of the National Academy of Sciences of the United States of America* 104, no. 26 (June 26, 2007): 11056–11061, https://doi.org/10.1073/pnas.0702413104; J. K. Zubieta, J. A. Bueller, L. R. Jackson, D. J. Scott, Y. Xu, R. A. Koeppe, T. E. Nichols, and C. S. Stohler, "Placebo Effects Mediated by Endogenous Opioid Activity on Mu-Opioid Receptors," *Journal of Neuroscience* 25, no. 34 (August 24, 2005): 7754–7762, https://doi.org/10.1523/JNEUROSCI.0439-05.2005.

6. J. D. Levine, N. C. Gordon, and H. L. Fields, "The Mechanism of Placebo Analgesia," *Lancet* 2, no. 8091 (September 23, 1978): 654–657, https://doi.org/10.1016/s0140-6736(78)92762-9.

7. M. Amanzio and F. Benedetti, "Neuropharmacological Dissection of Placebo Analgesia: Expectation-Activated Opioid Systems versus Conditioning

-Activated Specific Subsystems," *Journal of Neuroscience* 19, no. 1 (January 1 1999): 484–494, https://www.ncbi.nlm.nih.gov/pubmed/9870976.

8. Petrovic, Kalso, Petersson, and Ingvar, "Placebo and Opioid Analgesia."

9. F. Eippert, U. Bingel, E. D. Schoell, J. Yacubian, R. Klinger, J. Lorenz, and C. Buchel, "Activation of the Opioidergic Descending Pain Control System Underlies Placebo Analgesia," *Neuron* 63, no. 4 (August 27, 2009): 533–543, https://doi.org/10.1016/j.neuron.2009.07.014.

10. S. Geuter, L. Koban, and T. D. Wager, "The Cognitive Neuroscience of Placebo Effects: Concepts, Predictions, and Physiology," *Annual Review of Neuroscience* 40 (July 25, 2017): 167–188, https://doi.org/10.1146/annurev-neuro-072116-031132.

11. M. Lopez-Sola, S. Geuter, L. Koban, J. A. Coan, and T. D. Wager, "Brain Mechanisms of Social Touch-Induced Analgesia in Females," *Pain* 160, no. 9 (September 2019): 2072–2085, https://doi.org/10.1097/j.pain.0000000000001599; M. C. Reddan, H. Young, J. Falkner, M. Lopez-Sola, and T. D. Wager, "Touch and Social Support Influence Interpersonal Synchrony and Pain," *Social Cognitive and Affective Neuroscience* 15, no. 10 (November 10, 2020): 1064–1075, https://doi.org/10.1093/scan/nsaa048.

12. T. D. Wager and L. Y. Atlas, "The Neuroscience of Placebo Effects: Connecting Context, Learning and Health," *Nature Reviews Neuroscience* 16, no. 7 (July 2015): 403–418, https://doi.org/10.1038/nrn3976.

13. H. L. Fields, "Pain Modulation: Expectation, Opioid Analgesia and Virtual Pain," *Progress in Brain Research* 122 (2000): 245–253, https://doi.org/10.1016/s0079-6123(08)62143-3.

14. G. Westheimer, "Was Helmholtz a Bayesian?," *Perception* 37, no. 5 (2008): 642–650, https://doi.org/10.1068/p5973.

15. K. Friston, J. Kilner, and L. Harrison, "A Free Energy Principle for the Brain," *Journal of Physiology* (Paris) 100, no. 1–3 (July–September 2006): 70–87, https://doi.org/10.1016/j.jphysparis.2006.10.001.

16. A. Grahl, S. Onat, and C. Buchel, . "The Periaqueductal Gray and Bayesian Integration in Placebo Analgesia,"." *El eLife* 7 (Mar (March 20, 2018), . https://doi.org/10.7554/eLife.32930.

17. C. G. Goetz, J. Wuu, M. P. McDermott, C. H. Adler, S. Fahn, C. R. Freed, R. A. Hauser, et al., "Placebo Response in Parkinson's Disease: Comparisons among 11 Trials Covering Medical and Surgical Interventions," *Movement Disorders* 23, no. 5 (April 15, 2008): 690–699, https://doi.org/10.1002/mds.21894.

18. R. de la Fuente-Fernandez, T. J. Ruth, V. Sossi, M. Schulzer, D. B. Calne, and A. J. Stoessl, "Expectation and Dopamine Release: Mechanism of the Placebo Effect in Parkinson's Disease," *Science* 293, no. 5532 (August 10, 2001):

1164–1166, https://doi.org/10.1126/science.1060937; R. de la Fuente-Fernandez, A. G. Phillips, M. Zamburlini, V. Sossi, D. B. Calne, T. J. Ruth, and A. J. Stoessl, "Dopamine Release in Human Ventral Striatum and Expectation of Reward," *Behavioural Brain Research* 136, no. 2 (November 15, 2002): 359–363, https://doi.org/10.1016/s0166-4328(02)00130-4.

19. Wager and Atlas, "The Neuroscience of Placebo Effects."

20. A. Khan and W. A. Brown, "Antidepressants versus Placebo in Major Depression: An Overview," *World Psychiatry* 14, no. 3 (October 2015): 294–300, https://doi.org/10.1002/wps.20241.

21. H. S. Mayberg, J. A. Silva, S. K. Brannan, J. L. Tekell, R. K. Mahurin, S. McGinnis, and P. A. Jerabek, "The Functional Neuroanatomy of the Placebo Effect," *American Journal of Psychiatry* 159, no. 5 (May 2002): 728–737, https://doi.org/10.1176/appi.ajp.159.5.728.

22. M. Pecina, A. S. Bohnert, M. Sikora, E. T. Avery, S. A. Langenecker, B. J. Mickey, and J. K. Zubieta, "Association between Placebo-Activated Neural Systems and Antidepressant Responses: Neurochemistry of Placebo Effects in Major Depression," *JAMA Psychiatry* 72, no. 11 (November 2015): 1087–1094, https://doi.org/10.1001/jamapsychiatry.2015.1335; M. Pecina, M. Sikora, E. T. Avery, J. Heffernan, S. Pecina, B. J. Mickey, and J. K. Zubieta, "Striatal Dopamine D2/3 Receptor-Mediated Neurotransmission in Major Depression: Implications for Anhedonia, Anxiety and Treatment Response," *European Neuropsychopharmacology* 27, no. 10 (October 2017): 977–986, https://doi.org/10.1016/j.euroneuro.2017.08.427.

Chapter 4

1. S. Adler, *Sleep Paralysis: Night-Mares, Nocebos, and the Mind-Body Connection* (New Brunswick, NJ: Rutgers University Press, 2011).

2. N. Sawamoto, M. Honda, T. Okada, T. Hanakawa, M. Kanda, H. Fukuyama, J. Konishi, and H. Shibasaki, "Expectation of Pain Enhances Responses to Nonpainful Somatosensory Stimulation in the Anterior Cingulate Cortex and Parietal Operculum/Posterior Insula: An Event-Related Functional Magnetic Resonance Imaging Study," *Journal of Neuroscience* 20, no. 19 (October 1, 2000): 7438–7445, https://www.ncbi.nlm.nih.gov/pubmed/11007903; T. Koyama, J. G. McHaffie, P. J. Laurienti, and R. C. Coghill, "The Subjective Experience of Pain: Where Expectations Become Reality," *Proceedings of the National Academy of Sciences of the United States of America* 102, no. 36 (September 6, 2005): 12950–12955, https://doi.org/10.1073/pnas.0408576102; J. R. Keltner, A. Furst, C. Fan, R. Redfern, B. Inglis, and H. L. Fields, "Isolating the Modulatory Effect of Expectation on Pain Transmission: A Functional

Magnetic Resonance Imaging Study," *Journal of Neuroscience* 26, no. 16 (April 19, 2006): 4437–4443, https://doi.org/10.1523/JNEUROSCI.4463-05.2006.

3. P. M. Ridker, "The Jupiter Trial: Results, Controversies, and Implications for Prevention," *Circulation: Cardiovascular Quality and Outcomes* 2, no. 3 (May 2009): 279–285, https://doi.org/10.1161/CIRCOUTCOMES.109.868299.

4. F. A. Wood, J. P. Howard, J. A. Finegold, A. N. Nowbar, D. M. Thompson, A. D. Arnold, C. A. Rajkumar, et al., "N-of-1 Trial of a Statin, Placebo, or No Treatment to Assess Side Effects," *New England Journal of Medicine* 383, no. 22 (November 26, 2020): 2182–2184, https://doi.org/10.1056/NEJMc2031173.

5. M. Amanzio, L. L. Corazzini, L. Vase, and F. Benedetti, "A Systematic Review of Adverse Events in Placebo Groups of Anti-Migraine Clinical Trials," *Pain* 146, no. 3 (December 2009): 261–269, https://doi.org/10.1016/j.pain.2009.07.010; W. Rief, Y. Nestoriuc, A. von Lilienfeld-Toal, I. Dogan, F. Schreiber, S. G. Hofmann, A. J. Barsky, and J. Avorn, "Differences in Adverse Effect Reporting in Placebo Groups in SSRI and Tricyclic Antidepressant Trials: A Systematic Review and Meta-Analysis," *Drug Safety* 32, no. 11 (2009): 1041–1056, https://doi.org/10.2165/11316580-000000000-00000.

6. A. Silvestri, P. Galetta, E. Cerquetani, G. Marazzi, R. Patrizi, M. Fini, and G. M. Rosano, "Report of Erectile Dysfunction after Therapy with Beta-blockers Is Related to Patient Knowledge of Side Effects and Is Reversed by Placebo," *European Heart Journal* 24, no. 21 (November 2003): 1928–1932, https://doi.org/10.1016/j.ehj.2003.08.016.

7. T. J. Kaptchuk, J. M. Kelley, L. A. Conboy, R. B. Davis, C. E. Kerr, E. E. Jacobson, I. Kirsch, et al., "Components of Placebo Effect: Randomised Controlled Trial in Patients with Irritable Bowel Syndrome," *British Medical Journal* 336, no. 7651 (May 3, 2008): 999–1003, https://doi.org/10.1136/bmj.39524.439618.25.

8. L. C. Howe, J. P. Goyer, and A. J. Crum, "Harnessing the Placebo Effect: Exploring the Influence of Physician Characteristics on Placebo Response," *Health Psychology* 36, no. 11 (November 2017): 1074–1082, https://doi.org/10.1037/hea0000499.

9. H. E. Yetman, N. Cox, S. R. Adler, K. T. Hall, and V. E. Stone, "What Do Placebo and Nocebo Effects Have to Do with Health Equity? The Hidden Toll of Nocebo Effects on Racial and Ethnic Minority Patients in Clinical Care," *Frontiers in psychology* 12 (2021): 788230. https://doi.org/10.3389/fpsyg.2021.788230.

10. P. Friesen, and C. Blease, "Placebo Effects and Racial and Ethnic Health Disparities: An Unjust and Underexplored Connection," *Journal of Medical Ethics* 44, no. 11 (November 2018): 774–781, https://doi.org/10.1136/medethics-2018-104811.

11. E. M. Hooper, L. M. Comstock, J. M. Goodwin, and J. S. Goodwin, "Patient Characteristics That Influence Physician Behavior," *Medical Care* 20, no. 6 (June 1982): 630–638, https://doi.org/10.1097/00005650-198206000-00009.

12. W. J. Ferguson and L. M. Candib, "Culture, Language, and the Doctor-Patient Relationship," *Family Medicine* 34, no. 5 (May 2002): 353–361, https://www.ncbi.nlm.nih.gov/pubmed/12038717.

13. R. L. Johnson, D. Roter, N. R. Powe, and L. A. Cooper, "Patient Race/Ethnicity and Quality of Patient-Physician Communication during Medical Visits," *American Journal of Public Health* 94, no. 12 (December 2004): 2084–2090, https://doi.org/10.2105/ajph.94.12.2084.

14. L. Y. Atlas, "A Social Affective Neuroscience Lens on Placebo Analgesia," *Trends in Cognitive Sciences* 25, no. 11 (November 2021): 992–1005, https://doi.org/10.1016/j.tics.2021.07.016.

15. A. W. M. Evers, L. Colloca, C. Blease, J. Gaab, K. B. Jensen, L. Y. Atlas, C. J. Beedie, et al., "What Should Clinicians Tell Patients about Placebo and Nocebo Effects? Practical Considerations Based on Expert Consensus," *Psychotherapy and Psychosomatics* 90, no. 1 (2021): 49–56, https://doi.org/10.1159/000510738.

16. L. Colloca and A. J. Barsky, "Placebo and Nocebo Effects," *New England Journal of Medicine* 382, no. 6 (February 6, 2020): 554–561, https://doi.org/10.1056/NEJMra1907805.

17. D. L. Washington, J. Bowles, S. Saha, C. R. Horowitz, S. Moody-Ayers, A. F. Brown, V. E. Stone, et al., "Transforming Clinical Practice to Eliminate Racial-Ethnic Disparities in Healthcare," *Journal of General Internal Medicine* 23, no. 5 (May 2008): 685–691, https://doi.org/10.1007/s11606-007-0481-0.

18. Y. Sciama, "France Brings Back a Phased-Out Drug after Patients Rebel against Its Replacement," *ScienceInsider*, September 27, 2017, https://www.science.org/content/article/france-brings-back-phased-out-drug-after-patients-rebel-against-its-replacement.

19. K. Faasse, K., T. Cundy, and K. J. Petrie, "Thyroxine: Anatomy of a Health Scare," *British Medical Journal* 339 (December 29 2009): b5613, https://doi.org/10.1136/bmj.b5613.

20. M. Amanzio, J. Howick, M. Bartoli, G. E. Cipriani, and J. Kong, "How Do Nocebo Phenomena Provide a Theoretical Framework for the COVID-19 Pandemic?," *Frontiers in Psychology* 11 (2020): 589884, https://doi.org/10.3389/fpsyg.2020.589884.

21. J. W. Haas, F. L. Bender, S. Ballou, J. M. Kelley, M. Wilhelm, F. G. Miller, W. Rief, et al., "Frequency of Adverse Events in the Placebo Arms of COVID-19 Vaccine Trials: A Systematic Review and Meta-analysis," *JAMA Network*

Open 5, no. 1 (2022): e2143955, https://https://jamanetwork.com/journals/jamanetworkopen/fullarticle/2788172.

22. W. S. Chou and A. Budenz, "Considering Emotion in COVID-19 Vaccine Communication: Addressing Vaccine Hesitancy and Fostering Vaccine Confidence," *Health Communication* 35, no. 14 (December 2020): 1718–1722, https://doi.org/10.1080/10410236.2020.1838096.

23. "U.S. COVID-19 Vaccine Tracker: See Your State's Progress," 2021, https://www.mayoclinic.org/coronavirus-covid-19/vaccine-tracker; "COVID Data Tracker Weekly Review," Centers for Disease Control and Prevention, 2021, https://www.cdc.gov/coronavirus/2019-ncov/covid-data/covidview/index.html.

24. "COVID-19 19 Tracker," Reuters, 2021, https://graphics.reuters.com/world-coronavirus-tracker-and-maps/countries-and-territories/portugal/;
M. Santora and R. Minder, "In Portugal, There Is Virtually No One Left to Vaccinate," *New York Times*, 2021, https://www.nytimes.com/2021/10/01/world/europe/portugal-vaccination-rate.html.

Chapter 5

1. R. H. Dworkin, D. C. Turk, N. P. Katz, M. C. Rowbotham, S. Peirce-Sandner, I. Cerny, C. S. Clingman, et al., "Evidence-Based Clinical Trial Design for Chronic Pain Pharmacotherapy: A Blueprint for ACTION," *Pain* 152, no. 3 (March 2011): S107–S115, https://doi.org/10.1016/j.pain.2010.11.008; K. Evans, H. Romero, E. L. Spierings, and N. Katz, "The Relation between the Placebo Response, Observed Treatment Effect, and Failure to Meet Primary Endpoint: A Systematic Review of Clinical Trials of Preventative Pharmacological Migraine Treatments," *Cephalalgia* 41, no. 2 (February 2021): 247–255, https://doi.org/10.1177/0333102420960020.

2. O. J. Wouters, M. McKee, and J. Luyten, "Estimated Research and Development Investment Needed to Bring a New Medicine to Market, 2009–2018," *Journal of the American Medical Association* 323, no. 9 (March 3, 2020): 844–853, https://doi.org/10.1001/jama.2020.1166.

3. S. Pretorius and A. Grignolo, "Phase III Trial Failures: Costly, but Preventable," *Applied Clinical Trials* 25, no. 8 (2016), https://www.appliedclinicaltrialsonline.com/view/phase-iii-trial-failures-costly-preventable.

4. "2021 Alzheimer's Disease Facts and Figures: Race, Ethnicity and Alzheimer's in America," Alzheimer's Association, 2021, https://www.alz.org/media/documents/alzheimers-facts-and-figures.pdf.

5. F. Benedetti, C. Arduino, S. Costa, S. Vighetti, L. Tarenzi, I. Rainero, and G. Asteggiano, "Loss of Expectation-Related Mechanisms in Alzheimer's Disease

Makes Analgesic Therapies Less Effective," *Pain* 121, no. 1–2 (March 2006): 133–144, https://doi.org/10.1016/j.pain.2005.12.016.

6. J. Lim, L. Wang, N. Best, J. Liu, J. Yuan, F. Yong, L. Zhang, et al., "Reducing Patient Burden in Clinical Trials through the Use of Historical Controls: Appropriate Selection of Historical Data to Minimize Risk of Bias," *Therapeutic Innovation and Regulatory Science* 54, no. 4 (July 2020): 850–860, https://doi .org/10.1007/s43441-019-00014-4; K. Ito and K. Romero, "Placebo Effect in Subjects with Cognitive Impairment," *International Review of Neurobiology* 153 (2020): 213–230, https://doi.org/10.1016/bs.irn.2020.03.032.

7. J. Sevigny, P. Chiao, T. Bussiere, P. H. Weinreb, L. Williams, M. Maier, R. Dunstan, et al., "The Antibody Aducanumab Reduces Aβ Plaques in Alzheimer's Disease," *Nature* 537, no. 7618 (September 1, 2016): 50–56, https://doi .org/10.1038/nature19323.

8. R. K. McHugh, S. W. Whitton, A. D. Peckham, J. A. Welge, and M. W. Otto, "Patient Preference for Psychological vs Pharmacologic Treatment of Psychiatric Disorders: A Meta-Analytic Review," *Journal of Clinical Psychiatry* 74, no. 6 (June 2013): 595–602, https://doi.org/10.4088/JCP.12r07757.

9. I. Kirsch and G. Sapirstein, "Listening to Prozac but Hearing Placebo: A Meta-Analysis of Antidepressant Medication," *Prevention and Treatment* 1, no. 2 (1998), article 2a, https://psycnet.apa.org/record/1999-11094-001.

10. A. Khan, R. M. Leventhal, S. R. Khan, and W. A. Brown, "Severity of Depression and Response to Antidepressants and Placebo: An Analysis of the Food and Drug Administration Database," *Journal of Clinical Psychopharmacology* 22, no. 1 (February 2002): 40–45, https://www.ncbi.nlm.nih.gov /pubmed/11799341.

11. I. Kirsch, B. J. Deacon, T. B. Huedo-Medina, A. Scoboria, T. J. Moore, and B. T. Johnson, "Initial Severity and Antidepressant Benefits: A Meta-Analysis of Data Submitted to the Food and Drug Administration," *PLoS Medicine* 5, no. 2 (February 2008): e45, https://doi.org/10.1371/journal.pmed.0050045.

12. E. H. Turner, A. M. Matthews, E. Linardatos, R. A. Tell, and R. Rosenthal, "Selective Publication of Antidepressant Trials and Its Influence on Apparent Efficacy," *New England Journal of Medicine* 358, no. 3 (January 17, 2008): 252–260, https://doi.org/10.1056/NEJMsa065779.

13. A. Cipriani, T. A. Furukawa, G. Salanti, A. Chaimani, L. Z. Atkinson, Y. Ogawa, S. Leucht, et al., "Comparative Efficacy and Acceptability of 21 Antidepressant Drugs for the Acute Treatment of Adults with Major Depressive Disorder: A Systematic Review and Network Meta-Analysis," *Lancet* 391, no. 10128 (April 7, 2018): 1357–1366, https://doi.org/10.1016/S0140 -6736(17)32802-7.

14. M. Stone, S. N. Kalaria, K. Richardville, and B. J. Miller, "Components and Trends in Treatment Effects in Randomized Placebo-Controlled Trials in Major Depressive Disorder from 1979–2016" (paper presented at the American Society of Clinical Psychopharmacology Annual Conference, May 2018), https://www.researchgate.net/publication/334806796_Components_and_trends_in_treatment_effects_in_randomized_placebo-controlled_trials_in_major_depressive_disorder_from_1979-2016.

15. K. T. Hall, L. Vase, D. K. Tobias, H. T. Dashti, J. Vollert, T. J. Kaptchuk, and N. R. Cook, "Historical Controls in Randomized Clinical Trials: Opportunities and Challenges," *Clinical Pharmacology and Therapeutics* (June 30, 2020), https://doi.org/10.1002/cpt.1970.

16. J. R. Curtis, J. C. Larson, E. Delzell, M. A. Brookhart, S. M. Cadarette, R. Chlebowski, S. Judd, et al., "Placebo Adherence, Clinical Outcomes, and Mortality in the Women's Health Initiative Randomized Hormone Therapy Trials," *Medical Care* 49, no. 5 (May 2011): 427–435, https://doi.org/10.1097/MLR.0b013e318207ed9e.

17. T. R. Zijp, D. J. Touw, and J. F. M. van Boven, "User Acceptability and Technical Robustness Evaluation of a Novel Smart Pill Bottle Prototype Designed to Support Medication Adherence," *Patient Preference and Adherence* 14 (2020): 625–634, https://doi.org/10.2147/PPA.S240443.

18. S. Lee, J. R. Walker, L. Jakul, and K. Sexton, "Does Elimination of Placebo Responders in a Placebo Run-in Increase the Treatment Effect in Randomized Clinical Trials? A Meta-Analytic Evaluation," *Depression and Anxiety* 19, no. 1 (2004): 10–19, https://doi.org/10.1002/da.10134; T. A. Hulshof, S. U. Zuidema, C. C. Gispen-de Wied, and H. J. Luijendijk, "Run-in Periods and Clinical Outcomes of Antipsychotics in Dementia: A Meta-Epidemiological Study of Placebo-Controlled Trials," *Pharmacoepidemiology and Drug Safety* 29, no. 2 (February 2020): 125–133, https://doi.org/10.1002/pds.4903.

19. I. Chalmers and M. Clarke, "Commentary: The 1944 Patulin Trial: The First Properly Controlled Multicentre Trial Conducted under the Aegis of the British Medical Research Council," *International Journal of Epidemiology* 33, no. 2 (April 2004): 253–260, https://doi.org/10.1093/ije/dyh162.

20. Chalmers and Clarke, "Commentary."

Chapter 6

1. D. C. Sabiston and A. Blalock, "Experimental Ligation of the Internal Mammary Artery and Its Effect on Coronary Occlusion," *Surgery* 43, no. 6 (June 1958): 906–912, https://www.ncbi.nlm.nih.gov/pubmed/13543665.

2. L. A. Cobb, G. I. Thomas, D. H. Dillard, K. A. Merendino, and R. A. Bruce, "An Evaluation of Internal-Mammary-Artery Ligation by a Double-Blind Technic," *New England Journal of Medicine* 260, no. 22 (May 28, 1959): 1115–1118, https://doi.org/10.1056/NEJM195905282602204.

3. E. G. Dimond, C. F. Kittle, and J. E. Crockett, "Comparison of Internal Mammary Artery Ligation and Sham Operation for Angina Pectoris," *American Journal of Cardiology* 5 (April 1960): 483–486, https://doi.org/10.1016/0002-9149(60)90105-3.

4. H. K. Beecher, "Surgery as Placebo: A Quantitative Study of Bias," *Journal of the American Medical Association* 176 (July 1, 1961): 1102–1107, https://doi.org/10.1001/jama.1961.63040260007008.

5. H. K. Beecher, "Surgery as Placebo: A Quantitative Study of Bias," *Journal of the American Medical Association* 176 (July 1, 1961): 1102–1107, https://doi.org/10.1001/jama.1961.63040260007008.

6. Beecher, "Surgery as Placebo."

7. C. Linde, F. Gadler, L. Kappenberger, and L. Ryden, "Placebo Effect of Pacemaker Implantation in Obstructive Hypertrophic Cardiomyopathy. Pic Study Group. Pacing in Cardiomyopathy," *American Journal of Cardiology* 83, no. 6 (March 15, 1999): 903–907, https://doi.org/10.1016/s0002-9149(98)01065-0.

8. C. R. Freed, P. E. Greene, R. E. Breeze, W. Y. Tsai, W. DuMouchel, R. Kao, S. Dillon, et al., "Transplantation of Embryonic Dopamine Neurons for Severe Parkinson's Disease," *New England Journal of Medicine* 344, no. 10 (March 8, 2001): 710–719, https://doi.org/10.1056/NEJM200103083441002.

9. L. Wall, M. Hinwood, D. Lang, A. Smith, S. Bunzli, P. Clarke, P. F. M. Choong, et al., "Attitudes of Patients and Surgeons towards Sham Surgery Trials: A Protocol for a Scoping Review of Attributes to Inform a Discrete Choice Experiment," *British Medical Journal Open* 10, no. 3 (March 10, 2020): e035870, https://doi.org/10.1136/bmjopen 2019 035870.

10. J. B. Moseley, K. O'Malley, N. J. Petersen, T. J. Menke, B. A. Brody, D. H. Kuykendall, J. C. Hollingsworth, et al., "A Controlled Trial of Arthroscopic Surgery for Osteoarthritis of the Knee," *New England Journal of Medicine* 347, no. 2 (July 11, 2002): 81–88, https://doi.org/10.1056/NEJMoa013259.

11. T. L. N. Jarvinen and G. H. Guyatt, "Arthroscopic Surgery for Knee Pain: A Highly Questionable Practice without Supporting Evidence of Even Moderate Quality," *British Journal of Sports Medicine* 50, no. 23 (December 2016): 1426–1427, https://doi.org/10.1136/bmj.i3934rep.

12. H. C. Patel, C. Hayward, B. A. Ozdemir, S. D. Rosen, H. Krum, A. R. Lyon, D. P. Francis, and C. di Mario, "Magnitude of Blood Pressure Reduction in the Placebo Arms of Modern Hypertension Trials: Implications for Trials of Renal

Denervation," *Hypertension* 65, no. 2 (February 2015): 401–406, https://doi
.org/10.1161/HYPERTENSIONAHA.114.04640.

13. A. Persu, F. Maes, J. Renkin, and A. Pathak, "Renal Denervation in Hypertensive Patients: Back to Anatomy?," *Hypertension* 76, no. 4 (October 2020): 1084–1086, https://doi.org/10.1161/HYPERTENSIONAHA.120.15834.

14. K. Wartolowska, A. Judge, S. Hopewell, G. S. Collins, B. J. Dean, I. Rombach, D. Brindley, et al., "Use of Placebo Controls in the Evaluation of Surgery: Systematic Review," *British Medical Journal* 348 (May 21, 2014): g3253, https://doi.org/10.1136/bmj.g3253.

15. D. L. Bhatt, D. E. Kandzari, W. W. O'Neill, R. D'Agostino, J. M. Flack, B. T. Katzen, M. B. Leon, et al., "A Controlled Trial of Renal Denervation for Resistant Hypertension," *New England Journal of Medicine* 370, no. 15 (April 10, 2014): 1393–1401, https://doi.org/10.1056/NEJMoa1402670.

16. Jarvinen and Guyatt, "Arthroscopic Surgery for Knee Pain"; A. Carr, "Arthroscopic Surgery for Degenerative Knee," *British Medical Journal* 350 (2015): h2983, https://doi.org/10.1136/bmj.h2983.

Chapter 7

1. A. Kern, C. Kramm, C. M. Witt, and J. Barth, "The Influence of Personality Traits on the Placebo/Nocebo Response: A Systematic Review," *Journal of Psychosomatic Research* 128 (January 2020): 109866, https://doi.org/10.1016/j .jpsychores.2019.109866.

2. A. L. Geers, J. A. Wellman, S. L. Fowler, S. G. Helfer, and C. R. France, "Dispositional Optimism Predicts Placebo Analgesia," *Journal of Pain* 11, no. 11 (November 2010): 1165–1171, https://doi.org/10.1016/j.jpain.2010.02.014.

3. A. L. Geers, S. G. Helfer, K. Kosbab, P. E. Weiland, and S. J. Landry, "Reconsidering the Role of Personality in Placebo Effects: Dispositional Optimism, Situational Expectations, and the Placebo Response," *Journal of Psychosomatic Research* 58, no. 2 (February 2005): 121–127, https://www.ncbi.nlm.nih.gov /pubmed/15820839.

4. J. M. Kelley, A. J. Lembo, J. S. Ablon, J. J. Villanueva, L. A. Conboy, R. Levy, C. D. Marci, et al., "Patient and Practitioner Influences on the Placebo Effect in Irritable Bowel Syndrome," *Psychosomatic Medicine* 71, no. 7 (September 2009): 789–797, https://doi.org/10.1097/PSY.0b013e3181acee12.

5. P. Tetreault, A. Mansour, E. Vachon-Presseau, T. J. Schnitzer, A. V. Apkarian, and M. N. Baliki, "Brain Connectivity Predicts Placebo Response across Chronic Pain Clinical Trials," *PLoS Biology* 14, no. 10 (October 2016): e1002570, https://doi.org/10.1371/journal.pbio.1002570.

6. E. Vachon-Presseau, S. E. Berger, T. B. Abdullah, L. Huang, G. A. Cecchi, J. W. Griffith, T. J. Schnitzer, and A. V. Apkarian, "Brain and Psychological Determinants of Placebo Pill Response in Chronic Pain Patients," *Nature Communications* 9, no. 1 (September 12, 2018): article 3397, https://doi.org/10.1038/s41467-018-05859-1.

7. S. Zilcha-Mano, S. P. Roose, P. J. Brown, and B. R. Rutherford, "A Machine Learning Approach to Identifying Placebo Responders in Late-Life Depression Trials," *American Journal of Geriatric Psychiatry* 26, no. 6 (June 2018): 669–677, https://doi.org/10.1016/j.jagp.2018.01.001.

8. P. A. Nakonezny, T. L. Mayes, M. J. Byerly, and G. J. Emslie, "Predicting Placebo Response in Adolescents with Major Depressive Disorder: The Adolescent Placebo Impact Composite Score (APICS)," *Journal of Psychiatric Research* 68 (September 2015): 346–353, https://doi.org/10.1016/j.jpsychires.2015.05.003.

9. J. K. Park, S. H. Ahn, K. Shin, Y. J. Lee, Y. W. Song, and E. B. Lee, "Predictors of a Placebo Response in Patients with Hand Osteoarthritis: Post-Hoc Analysis of Two Randomized Controlled Trials," *BMC Musculoskeletal Disorders* 22, no. 1 (March 4, 2021): article 244, https://doi.org/10.1186/s12891-021-04089-9; J. Vollert, N. R. Cook, T. J. Kaptchuk, S. T. Sehra, D. K. Tobias, and K. T. Hall, "Assessment of Placebo Response in Objective and Subjective Outcome Measures in Rheumatoid Arthritis Clinical Trials," *Journal of the American Medical Association Network Open* 3, no. 9 (September 1, 2020): e2013196, https://doi.org/10.1001/jamanetworkopen.2020.13196.

10. J. Chen, B. K. Lipska, N. Halim, Q. D. Ma, M. Matsumoto, S. Melhem, B. S. Kolachana, et al., "Functional Analysis of Genetic Variation in Catechol-O-methyltransferase (COMT): Effects on mRNA, Protein, and Enzyme Activity in Postmortem Human Brain," *American Journal of Human Genetics* 75, no. 5 (November 2004): 807–821, https://doi.org/10.1086/425589.

11. K. T. Hall, A. J. Lembo, I. Kirsch, D. C. Ziogas, J. Douaiher, K. B. Jensen, L. A. Conboy, et al., "Catechol-O-methyltransferase val158met Polymorphism Predicts Placebo Effect in Irritable Bowel Syndrome," *PLoS One* 7, no. 10 (2012): e48135, https://doi.org/10.1371/journal.pone.0048135.

12. R.-S. Wang, A. J. Lembo, T. J. Kaptchuk, V. Cheng, J. Nee, J. Iturrino, M. Rao, J. Loscalzo, J. A. Silvester, and K. T. Hall, "Genomic Effects Associated with Response to Placebo Treatment in a Randomized Trial of Irritable Bowel Syndrome," *Frontiers in Pain Research* (2022), https://www.frontiersin.org/article/10.3389/fpain.2021.775386.

13. G. D. Slade, R. B. Fillingim, R. Ohrbach, H. Hadgraft, J. Willis, S. J. Arbes Jr., and I. E. Tchivileva, "COMT Genotype and Efficacy of Propranolol for TMD

Pain: A Randomized Trial," *Journal of Dental Research* 100, no. 2 (February 2021): 163–170, https://doi.org/10.1177/0022034520962733; K. T. Hall, J. Kossowsky, T. F. Oberlander, T. J. Kaptchuk, J. P. Saul, V. B. Wyller, E. Fagermoen, et al., "Genetic Variation in Catechol-O-methyltransferase Modifies Effects of Clonidine Treatment in Chronic Fatigue Syndrome," *Pharmacogenomics Journal* 16, no. 5 (October 2016): 454–460, https://doi.org/10.1038/tpj.2016.53; K. T. Hall, C. P. Nelson, R. B. Davis, J. E. Buring, I. Kirsch, M. A. Mittleman, J. Loscalzo, et al., "Polymorphisms in Catechol-O-methyltransferase Modify Treatment Effects of Aspirin on Risk of Cardiovascular Disease," *Arteriosclerosis, Thrombosis, and Vascular Biology* 34, no. 9 (September 2014): 2160–2167, https://doi.org/10.1161/ATVBAHA.114.303845; K. T. Hall, J. E. Buring, K. J. Mukamal, M. Vinayaga Moorthy, P. M. Wayne, T. J. Kaptchuk, E. M. Battinelli, et al., "COMT and Alpha-Tocopherol Effects in Cancer Prevention: Gene-Supplement Interactions in Two Randomized Clinical Trials," *Journal of the National Cancer Institute* 111, no. 7 (July 1, 2019): 684–694, https://doi.org/10.1093/jnci/djy204.

14. R. S. Wang, K. T. Hall, F. Giulianini, D. Passow, T. J. Kaptchuk, and J. Loscalzo, "Network Analysis of the Genomic Basis of the Placebo Effect," *JCI Insight* 2, no. 11 (June 2, 2017), https://doi.org/10.1172/jci.insight.93911.

Chapter 8

1. C. P. Skipper, K. A. Pastick, N. W. Engen, A. S. Bangdiwala, M. Abassi, S. M. Lofgren, D. A. Williams, et al., "Hydroxychloroquine in Nonhospitalized Adults with Early COVID-19: A Randomized Trial," *Annals of Internal Medicine* 173, no. 8 (October 20, 2020): 623–631, https://doi.org/10.7326/M20-4207.

2. L. R. Baden, H. M. El Sahly, B. Essink, K. Kotloff, S. Frey, R. Novak, D. Diemert, et al., "Efficacy and Safety of the mRNA-1273 SARS-CoV-2 Vaccine," *New England Journal of Medicine* 384, no. 5 (February 4, 2021): 403–416, https://doi.org/10.1056/NEJMoa2035389; J. H. Beigel, K. M. Tomashek, L. E. Dodd, A. K. Mehta, B. S. Zingman, A. C. Kalil, E. Hohmann, et al., "Remdesivir for the Treatment of Covid-19—Final Report," *New England Journal of Medicine* 383, no. 19 (November 5, 2020): 1813–1826, https://doi.org/10.1056/NEJMoa2007764.

3. J. Braga-Simoes, P. S. Costa, and J. Yaphe, "Placebo Prescription and Empathy of the Physician: A Cross-Sectional Study," *European Journal of General Practice* 23, no. 1 (December 2017): 98–104, https://doi.org/10.1080/13814788.2017.1291625; M. Fassler, K. Meissner, A. Schneider, and K. Linde, "Frequency and Circumstances of Placebo Use in Clinical Practice—a Systematic

Review of Empirical Studies," *BMC Medicine* 8 (February 23, 2010): article 15, https://doi.org/10.1186/1741-7015-8-15.

4. C. S. Harris, N. K. Campbell, and A. Raz, "Placebo Trends across the Border: US versus Canada," *PLoS One* 10, no. 11 (2015): e0142804, https://doi .org/10.1371/journal.pone.0142804.

5. P. C. Scriba, "Placeboaspekte der Arzt-Patienten-Beziehung. Übersicht" [Placebo and the relationship between doctors and patients. Overview]. *Bundesgesundheitsblatt Gesundheitsforschung Gesundheitsschutz* 55, no. 9 (September 2012): 1113–1117, https://doi.org/10.1007/s00103-012-1526-z.

6. T. J. Kaptchuk and F. G. Miller," "Open Label Placebo: Can Honestly Prescribed Placebos Evoke Meaningful Therapeutic Benefits?," *British Medical Journal* 363 (October 2, 2018): k3889, https://doi.org/10.1136/bmj.k3889.

7. C. Carvalho, J. M. Caetano, L. Cunha, P. Rebouta, T. J. Kaptchuk, and I. Kirsch, "Open-Label Placebo Treatment in Chronic Low Back Pain: A Randomized Controlled Trial," *Pain* 157, no. 12 (December 2016): 2766–2772, https://doi.org/10.1097/j.pain.0000000000000700; T. W. Hoenemeyer, T. J. Kaptchuk, T. S. Mehta, and K. R. Fontaine, "Open-Label Placebo Treatment for Cancer-Related Fatigue: A Randomized-Controlled Clinical Trial," *Scientific Reports* 8, no. 1 (February 9, 2018): article 2784, https://doi.org/10.1038 /s41598-018-20993-y; E. S. Zhou, K. T. Hall, A. L. Michaud, J. E. Blackmon, A. H. Partridge, and C. J. Recklitis, "Open-Label Placebo Reduces Fatigue in Cancer Survivors: A Randomized Trial," *Support Care Cancer* 27 (October 10, 2018): 2179–2187, https://doi.org/10.1007/s00520-018-4477-6; M. Schaefer, R. Harke, and C. Denke, "Open-Label Placebos Improve Symptoms in Allergic Rhinitis: A Randomized Controlled Trial," *Psychotherapy and Psychosomatics* 85, no. 6 (2016): 373–374, https://doi.org/10.1159/000447242; M. von Wernsdorff, M. L. Loef, B. Tuschen-Caffier, and S. Schmidt, "Effects of Open-Label Placebos in Clinical Trials: A Systematic Review and Meta-Analysis," *Scientific Reports* 11, no. 1 (February 16, 2021): article 3855, https://doi.org/10.1038 /s41598-021-83148-6.

8. G. Ongaro and T. J. Kaptchuk, "Symptom Perception, Placebo Effects, and the Bayesian Brain," *Pain* 160, no. 1 (January 2019): 1–4, https://doi. org/10.1097/j.pain.0000000000001367.

9. S. H. Kollins, D. J. DeLoss, E. Canadas, J. Lutz, R. L. Findling, R. S. E. Keefe, J. N. Epstein, et al., "A Novel Digital Intervention for Actively Reducing Severity of Paediatric ADHD (STARS-ADHD): A Randomised Controlled Trial," *Lancet Digital Health* 2, no. 4 (April 2020): e168–e178, https://doi.org/10.1016 /S2589-7500(20)30017-0.

10. P. Cipresso, I. A. C. Giglioli, M. A. Raya, and G. Riva, "The Past, Present, and Future of Virtual and Augmented Reality Research: A Network and Cluster Analysis of the Literature," *Frontiers in Psychology* 9 (2018): 2086, https://doi.org/10.3389/fpsyg.2018.02086.

11. M. J. Park, D. J. Kim, U. Lee, E. J. Na, and H. J. Jeon, "A Literature Overview of Virtual Reality (VR) in Treatment of Psychiatric Disorders: Recent Advances and Limitations," *Frontiers in Psychiatry* 10 (2019): 505, https://doi.org/10.3389/fpsyt.2019.00505; Z. Trost, C. France, M. Anam, and C. Shum, "Virtual Reality Approaches to Pain: Toward a State of the Science," *Pain* 162, no. 2 (February 1, 2021): 325–331, https://doi.org/10.1097/j.pain.0000000000002060.

12. J. R. Forsyth, H. Chase, N. W. Roberts, L. C. Armitage, and A. J. Farmer, "Application of the National Institute for Health and Care Excellence Evidence Standards Framework for Digital Health Technologies in Assessing Mobile-Delivered Technologies for the Self-Management of Type 2 Diabetes Mellitus: Scoping Review," *JMIR Diabetes* 6, no. 1 (February 16, 2021): e23687, https://doi.org/10.2196/23687.

FURTHER READING

Adler, Shelley R. *Sleep Paralysis*. New Brunswick, NJ: Rutgers University Press, 2011.

Benedetti, Fabrizio. *Placebo Effects*. Oxford: Oxford University Press, 2014.

Colloca, Luana, ed. *Neurobiology of the Placebo Effect, Part I*. Cambridge, MA: Academic Press, 2018.

Colloca, Luana, Magne Arve Flaten, and Karin Meissner, eds. *Placebo and Pain: From Bench to Bedside*. Oxford: Elsevier, 2013.

Cramp, Arthur Joseph. *Nostrums and Quackery and Pseudo-Medicine*. Vol. 1. Chicago: Press of American Medical Association, 1912.

Evans, Dylan. *Placebo: Mind over Matter in Modern Medicine*. New York: Oxford University Press, 2004.

Fish, Jefferson M. *Placebo Therapy: A Practical Guide to Social Influence in Psychotherapy*. San Francisco: Jossey-Bass, 1973.

Frank, Jerome D., and Julia B. Frank. *Persuasion and Healing: A Comparative Study of Psychotherapy*. Baltimore: Johns Hopkins University Press, 1993.

Harrington, Anne, ed. *The Placebo Effect: An Interdisciplinary Exploration*. Cambridge, MA: Harvard University Press, 1997.

Humphrey, Nicholas. "Great Expectations: The Evolutionary Psychology of Faith-Healing and the Placebo Response." In *Psychology at the Turn of the Millennium: Vol. 2: Social, Developmental, and Clinical Perspectives*, edited by Claes von Hofsten and Lars Bäckman, 225–246. Hove, UK: Psychology Press, 2002.

Lipton, Bruce H. *The Biology of Belief: Unleashing the Power of Consciousness, Matter and Miracles*. Carlsbad, CA: Hay House, 2016.

Moerman, Daniel. *Meaning, Medicine and the "Placebo Effect."* Cambridge: Cambridge University Press, 2002.

INDEX

DR. KATHRYN HALL is the Deputy Executive Director for Population Health and Health Equity at the Boston Public Health Commission. She is also a part-time Assistant Professor in the Division of Preventive Medicine and Director of Basic and Translation Research at Osher Center for Integrative Medicine at Brigham and Women's Hospital and Harvard Medical School.